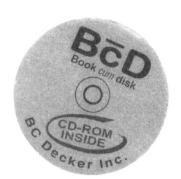

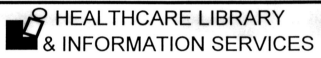

HEALTHCARE LIBRARY
& INFORMATION SERVICES

SCARBOROUGH & NORTH EAST YORKSHIRE HEALTHCARE NHS TRUST and
THE DEPARTMENT OF HEALTH SCIENCES, UNIVERSITY OF YORK (SCARBOROUGH SITE)
Scarborough Hospital, Woodlands Drive, Scarborough, North Yorkshire YO12 6QL
Telephone 01723 368111, extension 2075, Fax 01723 342018, Direct Line 01723 342184

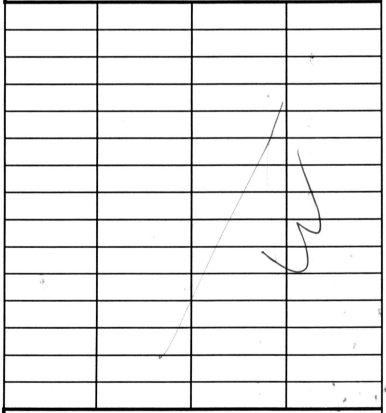

When returning books to the library, please place them
in the Returned Book Box.   No responsibility can be
accepted for books left elsewhere.

Evidence-Based

Family Medicine

Evidence-Based

Family

Medicine

Walter W. Rosser, M.D., CCFP, FCFP, MRCGP (UK)
Department of Family and Community Medicine
University of Toronto
Toronto, Ontario

M. Sharon Shafir, M.D., M.Ed., CCFP, FCFP
Department of Family and Community Medicine
University of Toronto
Toronto, Ontario

1998
B.C. Decker Inc.
Hamilton • London

B.C. Decker Inc.
4 Hughson Street South
P.O. Box 620, L.C.D. 1
Hamilton, Ontario L8N 3K7
Tel: 905-522-7017
Fax: 905-522-7839
e-mail: info@bcdecker.com
website: http://www.bcdecker.com

97 98 99 00 01 / BP / 9 8 7 6 5 4 3 2 1
Printed in Canada
ISBN 1-55009-053-4

Sales and Distribution

United States
Blackwell Science Inc.
Commerce Place
350 Main Street
Malden, MA 02148
U.S.A.
Tel: 1-800-215-1000

U.K., Europe, Scandinavia, Middle East
Blackwell Science Ltd.
c/o Marston Book Services Ltd.
P.O. Box 87
Oxford OX2 0DT
England
Tel: 44-1865-79115

Canada
B.C. Decker Inc.
4 Hughson Street South
P.O. Box 620, L.C.D. 1
Hamilton, Ontario L8N 3K7
Tel: 905-522-7017
Fax: 905-522-7839
e-mail: info@bcdecker.com

Australia
Blackwell Science Pty, Ltd.
54 University Street
Carlton, Victoria 3053
Australia
Tel: 03 9347 0300
Fax: 03 9349 3016

Japan
Igaku-Shoin Ltd.
Tokyo International P.O. Box 5063
1-28-36 Hongo, Bunkyo-ku
Tokyo 113, Japan
Tel: 3 3817 5680
Fax: 3 3815 7805

India
Jaypee Brothers Medical Publishers Ltd.
B-3 EMCA House, 23/23
Ansari Road, Daryaganj,
P.B. 7193, New Delhi – 110002, India
Tel: 11 3272143
Fax: 11 3276490

Notice: The authors and publisher have made every effort to ensure that the patient care recommended herein, including choice of drugs and drug dosages, is in accord with the accepted standard and practice at the time of publication. However, since research and regulation constantly change clinical standards, the reader is urged to check the product information sheet included in the package of each drug, which includes recommended doses, warnings, and contraindications. This is particularly important with new or infrequently used drugs.

Contents

Foreword

The head long rush to specialization in medical practice, teaching, and research that has characterized the United States, Germany, and other countries for the past 70 years was never fully embraced by many other nations, including Canada. An overcommitment to medical subspecialization and hospital-based care is presently in the midst of mitigation, based on a worldwide renaissance of primary care, driven largely by concerns about unsustainable costs of medical care. The value of primary care has been recognized again, and the contest for its survival has been fought and settled in favor of primary care as an essential foundation in effective health care systems. If this period of neglect and struggle were called Era One of primary care, we have entered without pause or respite into Era Two. This book is about Era Two.

In Era One, many primary care clinicians recognized that the discipline was not a summation of subsets of subspeciality knowledge. Experienced family doctors are widely known to alter their practice to accommodate the burden of suffering actually experienced by their patients, and primary care clinicians often struggle with the apparent discrepancies between what they were taught and the realities of daily practice. Now that there is a place under the sun for primary care, the challenge of Era Two is not existence, but superior performance. *Evidence-Based Family Medicine* is a bridge to Era Two for primary care clinicians, teachers, and their patients.

This text explains the intellectual basis of much of what goes wrong when knowledge is misapplied in primary care. Rather than lamenting this unfortunate circumstance, this text advances into Era Two with practical alternatives to improve primary care practice. Focusing on the questions that dominate the daily lives of family doctors and their patients, this text demonstrates a systematic approach to evaluating evidence and applying it to the benefit of people. Technical aspects of assessing evidence are made subservient to what matters to people. The elusive web of causality is embraced, rather than crammed into simplistic linear thinking. Building on the pivotal primary care concept of a sustained partnership between clinician and patients, the proposed Physician-Patient Partnership Papers offer tools for application today in practice that unite what is known with the values and preferences of patients.

This is a text for the primary care clinician who wants to know and assess the evidence that undergirds her/his practice. It is also a valuable resource for the tutor and teacher of those students and residents who need to understand primary care and its distinct challenges. It may be a text that promotes peace at the frayed boundaries of primary care and subspecialty care. Essentially, it is a light shining into Era Two of family medicine and primary care revealing important opportunities to improve primary care practice to the benefit of many individuals, one at a time.

April 1997

Larry Green, MD
Chair, Department of Family Medicine
University of Colorado Medical School
University of Colorado
Denver, Colorado USA

Preface

Until the middle of the 19th century, most interventions in clinical practice were based on the experience of generations of physicians. The evolution of epidemiology, and subsequently clinical epidemiology, resulted in methods that allowed the objective critique of therapies used in clinical practice. Multicentered, randomized trials now make it possible to answer fundamental questions about common medical interventions. The practice of evidence-based medicine requires an understanding of clinical epidemiology, as well as excellent communication skills, patience, and a commitment to provide the patient with the knowledge required to make informed choices.

Commercial interests often create perceptions of the necessity for a medical intervention. These perceptions may not be based on current scientific evidence, thereby creating dissonance between the patient and the physician trying to practice evidence-based medicine. The process of providing the patient with evidence-based information for decision making includes confirmation that the patient understands all risks and/or benefits of any intervention. In aid of this process, we have developed a practical model that is grounded in a theoretical understanding of the doctor-patient relationship in family and general practice. We hope that the time barriers encountered in family and general practice will be overcome through use of the Physician-Patient Partnership Papers (PPPPs) provided in the book.

The purpose of this book is to help present and future physicians, educators, and patients gain the knowledge and skills required to teach, practice, and use evidence-based medicine. To achieve this goal, the book has been divided into two sections. The first section consists of thirteen chapters outlining the basic skills and knowledge required to teach and learn about critically assessing the medical literature. The second section emphasizes the practical application of critical thinking to the clinical encounter in family and general practice, and includes a literature review written for patients, the references, and recommendations from organizations that base guidelines on critical reviews of the literature.

It is our hope that this book will move physicians and patients closer to the ideal of making as many medical management decisions as possible using appropriate and clinically relevant critically appraised evidence.

Toronto, Canada   W.W. Rosser
September 1997   M.S. Shafir

Acknowledgements

The authors would like to acknowledge the parts played by many others—Dr Larry Green for the Foreword; Dr Ian McWhinney for his review and comments on the manuscript; and for their critique and advice of specific sections, Drs Lorne Becker, Anne Biringer, June Carroll, Larry Culpepper, Mike Evans, Bernard Ewigman, Rick Glazier, Tony Graham, Gordon Hardacre, Gwen Jantz, Diane Kerbal, Cheryl Levitt, Eric Letovsky, Warren McIsaac, Graham Owen, and Yves Talbot. We especially want to acknowledge the part played by Dr John Frank in planting the seed out of which the PPPP grew.

For the time necessary to produce the draft manuscript Dr Rosser acknowledges the support of the University of Toronto and Dr Aberman, Dean, Faculty of Medicine, in granting a six-month study leave.

We have both greatly appreciated the support of family, friends and colleagues, and the patient support of Diane Dent and the staff at Decker.

PART I

Teaching and Learning Critical Thinking
in Family and General Practice

CHAPTER 1

Finding Published Evidence Relevant to Clinical Practice

———•—•———

Finding useful clinical information in the 1990s is like finding a special
grain of sand in a four meter tidal wave as it crashes onto the beach.
Anonymous

It is impossible to review even a small portion of the massive volume of medical literature published monthly. This chapter is designed to aid practitioners in finding useful information in the literature and to improve or develop a preliminary sorting strategy. Subsequent chapters provide the physician with sorting strategies for specific topics. Key terms introduced in this chapter are randomized trial, controlled trial, power calculations, empirical data, descriptive report, case-control study, cohort study, bias, meta-analysis, POEM and DOE. Consult the glossary for definitions.

LEARNING OBJECTIVES

Upon completion of this chapter the reader should be able to

1. determine the usefulness of medical information;
2. develop a systematic approach to determining what should or should not be read; and
3. use the learned strategies to assist with the selection of medical literature that provides evidence for clinical practice.

CHOOSING AN INFORMATION SOURCE

The MEDLINE[1] database of the National Library of Medicine contains 6,000,000 references from 4000 journals, with approximately 400,000 new entries added each year.[2] Currently, there are 19,304 articles on the subject of prostate neoplasm alone. It is estimated that a practitioner would need to read 6000 articles per day to keep up with everything important in the medical field.[2]

The sources of medical information available continue to increase as the "information highway"—the Internet with its thousands of web sites—evolves.

The first step in facing this overwhelming challenge is to determine how to sort the information presently used. Do not feel embarrassed or guilty for not having considered this concept, as most physicians do not have an organized strategy for sorting the literature. The simplest way to begin is to ask: What journals do I presently read or scan? How do I choose which journals I read? How do I decide which abstracts or articles to read? Have I developed a system for identifying articles that are important or relevant in the clinical setting?

If you have criteria to help select the information sources you regularly review including computerized guidelines, CME programs, medical newspapers and other print material, you will eliminate over 99% of all available information. Given the magnitude of this first-level sorting, the selection strategy deserves careful consideration.

Peer-Reviewed Versus Non-Peer-Reviewed Literature

Information published in sources other than medical journals should be considered non-peer-reviewed, unless convincingly demonstrated otherwise. An increasing number of medical journals are published without peer review, often under pharmaceutical company sponsorship; a healthy dose of scepticism is required when reading material from these sources. Journals such as *Canadian Family Physician*, *The Journal of Family Practice*, and *The British Journal of General Practice*, have a mixture of peer-reviewed articles and solicited review articles. These journals clearly identify the category into which each article falls. *The New England Journal of Medicine*, *Journal of the American Medical Association*, *British Medical Journal*, and *The Lancet* are examples of internationally recognized peer-reviewed journals. The pedigree of the journal in which a study is published does not guarantee the value of the study results for patients; however, these elite publications demand consideration as they are often quoted in local newspapers. There is a considerable body of literature critiquing the peer-review process and its dependence on two or three reviewers, who may bring their own biases to the reviews. Articles appearing in any journal, even peer-reviewed, should be critically assessed by the reader.

The Authors

Knowledge of the authors and their previous work on a topic may occasionally influence readers to select an article for reading.

Abstracts

Journals present abstracts for articles in different forms. Many journals are adopting a standard structured abstract format. This style of abstract allows one to be more efficient in judging the value of an article. A structured abstract consists of concise summaries under headings that include:

Objectives   The study objectives should be clearly stated. Absence of a clearly defined question suggests that the results will be of little value.

Method   Although much of the information and many of the procedures followed in medicine have not been rigorously assessed, the emphasis in evidence-based medicine is to ensure that an increasing percentage of medical interventions are based on high-quality evidence. The methods should be so clearly and transparently described that the study could be reproduced on the basis of that description. For family and general practitioners the description of the study population used in the trial is an important part of the methods section. Many clinical trials are conducted in tertiary care referral practices or hospitals, making the results of questionable value to family and general practitioners. The lack of good methodology may signal that further consideration of the study is not indicated.

Given the importance of study methods, a brief review of different study designs is presented.

Empirical   The weakest methodology is empirical knowledge, or "expert" opinion, commonly expressed in the hallways of hospitals or clinics and too frequently appearing in the pages of medical journals and newspapers. Opinions or observations from experience are not subjected to critical review. One should be reluctant to change practice strategies on the basis of empirical evidence alone.

Descriptive reports   In the past, physicians commonly published either individual case studies or a series of case studies about specific problems. Surgeons commonly publish a series of 10 or 20 cases when describing their experience and results. This type of descriptive study provides the basis from which a hypothesis can be generated to develop more rigorous trials. Conclusions drawn from a case series are only marginally stronger in quality than those drawn from purely empirical evidence.

Case-control studies   A case-control study is often used to determine the cause of a disease. The medical records of individuals with a disease are matched with medical records of individuals who have similar characteristics, such as age and gender, but who do not have the disease. An example of such a study is when people with heart disease are matched to people without heart disease and the cholesterol curves in each group are compared in an attempt to establish a relationship. Inferences and conclusions are often drawn from case-control studies, but the methodology is weak because of the many uncontrolled variables that exist in attempting to match individual characteristics. Bias is a major problem in these studies as researchers attempt to demonstrate a specific result.

Cohort study   The cohort study differs from a case-control study in that two or more groups of people are assembled and followed prospectively. For example, a cohort of patients with a number of important risk factors for cardiovascular diseases are assembled simultaneously with a control cohort of individuals who do not have these risk factors. Both groups are followed prospectively for a period of time before outcomes are determined. There is potential for bias in selection using the prospective method, but it is lower than that of retrospective case-control studies.

Randomized controlled trials   The strongest methodology is the randomized controlled trial (RCT) where patients, at the time of entry into the trial, are randomly allocated to either an "intervention" or "control" group. Large numbers of people are required to establish statistically significant differences between the two groups. Denying therapy to those in the control group, even if the therapy is not yet proven to be of benefit, may be considered unethical. Years or even decades of patient follow-up may be required to determine if the intervention provided a benefit. All of these factors make RCT studies difficult and expensive so that it is often impractical to carry out trials that can answer important practice-related questions (for further discussion see Chapter 5).

Meta-analysis   Meta-analysis is the methodology by which the results of a number of studies asking the same question and using similar methods are combined to increase their statistical power so that a more definite conclusion may be drawn. The best meta-analyses use randomized controlled trials (see Chapter 10).

Results   The results section of an abstract should provide the actual numbers of participants, dosages, etc., and provide the relevant statistical analyses. These results should be presented as a summary which clearly states the study's most important findings.

Conclusions   The conclusions in an abstract should be specific, answer the question posed by the study, and clearly reflect and link the objectives and results sections.

Other Strategies for Sorting Relevant from Irrelevant Literature

Many family physicians find it useful to seek out widely quoted or publicized articles and critically assess their clinical relevance. The media frequently misinterpret study results, or the results may apply only to a select population. This strategy helps to answer the patient's questions in an evidence-based way.

Conducting a literature search using a software package such as Grateful Med® to answer specific clinical questions is another approach to obtaining relevant information. Physicians need not be intimidated by the idea of doing a literature search using a computer software package; usually within 5 to 10 minutes one can complete a literature search using Grateful Med® and have the information needed for a reasonable answer to a question, even if not computer literate.[3] When requesting searches from a librarian, or doing the search personally, asking for abstracts will allow rapid selection of articles of value.

STORING USEFUL INFORMATION

Many physicians tear articles from medical journals and keep them in files listed according to specific conditions. One simple filing method is the International Classification of Health Problems in Primary Care (ICHPPC).[4] Its use will allow the accumulation of literature by problem, making it simpler to review the literature when that problem presents in the clinical setting. A "tear-out" file is also useful for clinical teaching to provide students and patients with relevant information. Alternatively, one can keep a computer file. Computer software packages are available that make classification and storage of references relatively simple.

DETERMINING THE USEFULNESS OF MEDICAL INFORMATION: POEM AND DOE

A formula for determining the usefulness of medical information for family physicians has been developed by Shaughnessy et al.[5] The formula is as follows:

Usefulness of Medical Information = Relevancy x Validity/Work Factor

This formula summarizes the needs of family and general practitioners who are interested in knowing how to help patients to a) live longer; b) function as closely as possible to their full capacity; c) have the highest level of life satisfaction as possible; and d) to be as pain- and symptom-free as possible.

The ultimate question the physician must ask is: Will the patient come closer to achieving all of these goals as a result of the proposed intervention?

TYPES OF EVIDENCE: POEM AND DOE

A study addressing quality of life issues, mortality, and morbidity is called a POEM, for *p*atient *o*riented *e*vidence that *m*atters. Studies classified as POEMs deal with patient outcomes and may lead physicians to alter their patterns of practice.[5] A study addressing factors such as organ function or biochemical levels in the blood deals with *d*isease *o*riented *e*vidence and is called a DOE. Our knowledge and understanding of etiology, prevalence, and pathophysiology, is enhanced by the DOE study. Asking the question, Is this article a POEM or a DOE? is fundamental and is emphasized throughout this book.

A great deal of the medical literature focuses on DOE studies. An example of a DOE study (one which deals with changes in organ systems, blood levels, or investigative procedures) can be drawn from the cholesterol debate, which also illustrates the fundamental difference in the approach to patients used by family physicians and specialists.

The cardiologist focuses on the effect of cholesterol-lowering agents and their impact on the LDL or serum cholesterol, and the reduction of cardiac event rates. These changes are DOE, although one could argue that a reduction of cardiac event rates falls between a POEM and a DOE. In contrast, the family and general practitioner is focused on longevity and quality of life and, in jargon, "all-cause mortality" (POEM). The cardiologist may advocate the use of various cholesterol-lowering agents, while the family and general practitioner remains somewhat ambivalent about these interventions, awaiting firm evidence of benefit to longevity. Although many of the cholesterol-lowering agents show a significant benefit for the reduction of cardiac event rates, only one agent has shown improvement in all-cause mortality for primary prevention.

Table 1–1 provides a series of examples of POEM outcomes, outcomes of studies that would be intermediate between a POEM and a DOE, and study outcomes on the same topic that would be DOE.

FURTHER AIDS FOR THE OVERWHELMED PHYSICIAN

The physician may justifiably ask the question: How practical is it for me to review the relevant literature? Reviewing more than three to six journals is an impossible task. Fortunately, a growing number of alternative strategies are being developed to help the physician deal with the increasing amount of available information. Two organizations that provide the family and general practitioner with excellent assistance include the Canadian Task Force on the Periodic Health Examination (which was established in 1976) and the Cochrane Collaboration.[6–8]

The Task Force on the Periodic Health Examination, funded by the Government of Canada, was created specifically to deal with the huge demand for tests, interventions, and medication continually emerging from the commercially driven American health care market. With free-flowing communication across the world's longest undefended border, there was a need to assess, in an objective way, what procedures are justifiable in a publicly funded health care system.[7] To meet this challenge, the Task Force developed a "transparent" method of critically appraising the literature on an intervention, classifying the quality of the evidence and assigning a rating from A to E. An A rating is given when there is firm evidence that the intervention is justified (using data from one or more RCTs); a B rating indicates that there is some evidence supporting the intervention; a C rating is given when there is insufficient evidence to either recommend the use or nonuse of the intervention; a D rating indicates that there is some evidence that the intervention is harmful; and E is given when there is firm evidence that the intervention will cause more harm than good.[7]

Recently, the Task Force consolidated 15 years of its work into a single volume entitled *The Canadian Guide to Clinical Preventive Health Care*,[7] affectionately known as "the brick," in reference to its size. Each chapter contains a detailed review and critique of the current literature regarding one or more preventive questions, and concludes with a recommendation regarding the value of the intervention (A to E). We believe that a copy of this book belongs in the office of every family and general practitioner attempting to practice evidence-based medicine. A similar book has been produced by the U.S. Preventive Services Task Force and also deserves consideration.[9]

The second important initiative, the Cochrane Collaboration, is named after the founding sponsor, Archie Cochrane, a British epidemiologist. The Cochrane Collaboration is a worldwide network of health care professionals and laypersons concerned with identifying, collecting, and analyzing literature that meets rigorous quality standards. The organization

Table 1–1   Examples of POEM vs DOE

	POEM	*Intermediate*	*DOE*
Cholesterol lowering	Improved all-cause mortality	Reduced cardiac events	Lower serum cholesterol
Reducing atherosclerotic plaques	Improved all-cause mortality	Reduced frequency of angina episodes	Improved cardiac blood flow on angiogram
Consuming a low-fat diet	Improved life expectancy	Improved self-esteem	Lower serum cholesterol
Hormone replacement therapy	Improved life expectancy and quality	Reduced risk of fractures	Increased bone density

TEACHING / LEARNING TIPS

- Select a variety of journals that individuals in your group read. Have each person time how long it takes to scan a journal, then describe the way in which they decide on the value of an article.

- Take a pile of articles and, as quickly as possible, classify each as POEM or DOE.

- Record the percentage of articles in each journal that have the potential to alter your pattern of practice (POEM).

- Take a series of articles and, as quickly as possible, classify them by the methodology used. It should be possible to do this by reading the abstract.

- Discuss what methods individuals in the group use to choose which journals they read.

- Discuss what methods individuals use to store information.

- Ask each group member to bring one journal that they read, discuss why they read it, and have others scan that journal to identify what they would read.

- Identify an article receiving extensive publicity and determine if it is relevant to your practice.

- Conduct a literature search on a topic of interest and, using abstracts, determine what percentage of identified literature is useful in answering the question.

- Alone, or with colleagues/students, assemble 6 to 10 recently published journals and rapidly review each, recording how many abstracts are fully read, partially read, or unread, and how many full articles individuals would read based on the abstract review. Discuss how each decision was made.

was formed by developing a large number of groups, each of which reviews a topic using specific and transparent methods. These efforts result in a constantly expanding database of high quality literature reviews, called the Cochrane Library, which is accessible to physicians worldwide.[8] Physicians, nurses, allied health professionals, and laypersons may join a working group of the Cochrane Collaboration and participate in the development of this important database. Since the Collaboration involves all medical disciplines it will continually pressure the medical profession towards the practice of evidence-based medicine.

One of the early products to emerge from the U.K. as the Collaboration was developing was a book entitled *A Guide to Effective Care in Pregnancy and Childbirth* by Enkin, Keirse, and Chalmers.[9] An earlier book, also using an evidence-based strategy, was titled *Primary Medical Care of Children and Adolescents* by Feldman, Rosser, and McGrath.[10] These books are examples of textbooks written in an evidence-based style. Journals such as *Canadian Family Physician* are incorporating articles written in a similar manner.

QUESTIONS TO ASK WHEN REVIEWING THE LITERATURE

1. Is the title interesting?
2. Is the outcome of the study a POEM or a DOE?
3. Do you know of the author? Does the author have a good reputation?
4. Is the abstract structured?
5. Does the study population correspond to your practice population?
6. What method is described to answer the research question?

RECOMMENDED READING

Department of Clinical Epidemiology, McMaster University. How to Read Medical Journals: (1) Why to read them and how to start reading them critically. Can Med Assoc J 1981;124(5):555–558.

Oxman AD, Sackett DL, Guyatt GH. Users' guide to the medical literature: 1. How to get started. JAMA 1993;270:2093–2095.

REFERENCES

1. ARNDTKA Information access in medicine. Overview: Relevance to dermatology and strategies for coping. Arch Dermatol 1992;128:1249–1256.

2. National Library of Medicine, Bethesda, MD: Medline 1997.

3. Haynes RB, Johnston ME, McKibbon KA, Walker CJ. A randomized controlled trial of a program to enhance clinical use of Medline. Online J of Current Clinical Trials 1993; Document No.56.

4. Lamberts H, Woods M. International Classification of Health Problems in Primary Care. Oxford: Oxford University Press, 1992.

5. Shaughnessy AF, Slawson DC, Bennet JH. Becoming an information master: A guidebook to the medical information jungle. J Fam Pract 1994;39:484–499.

6. Canadian Task Force on the Periodic Health Examination. The Periodic Health Examination. Can Med Assoc J 1979;121:1193–1254.

7. The Canadian Task Force on the Periodic Health Examination. The Canadian Guide to Clinical Preventive Health Care. Minister of Supply and Services Ottawa, Canada, 1994.

9. Report of the U.S. Preventive Services Task Force. Guide to Clinical Preventive Services. Baltimore: Williams and Wilkins, 1989.

8. Oxman A, Chalmers I, Clarke EM, et al. Cochrane Collaboration Handbook. Oxford: Cochrane Collaboration, 1994.

9. Enkin M, Keirse J, Chalmers I. A Guide to Effective Care in Pregnancy and Childbirth. Oxford: Oxford University Press, 1988.

10. Feldman W, Rosser W, McGrath P. Primary Medical Care of Children and Adolescents. New York: Oxford University Press, 1987.

CHAPTER 2

Using Two-by-Two Tables to Assess Diagnostic Tests

"It is a test of true theories not only to account for but to predict phenomena."
William Whewell 1794–1886

Understanding the *concept* of the two-by-two table is fundamental to understanding how to critique the medical literature. Understanding the *principles* and the *terminology* of the two-by-two table is essential for the teaching and practice of evidence-based medicine. An understanding of the terms specificity, sensitivity, positive predictive value, negative predictive value, gold standard, and blinding, is necessary to fully understand this chapter. Consult the glossary for definitions.

LEARNING OBJECTIVES

Upon completion of this chapter, the reader should be able to:
1. understand the terminology used in discussion of the two-by two table;
2. calculate the specificity, sensitivity and positive predictive value of a diagnostic test;
3. apply the principles of the two-by-two table when making decisions regarding the value of diagnostic tests in the clinical setting; and
4. incorporate teaching of the two-by-two table into his/her clinical or educational environment.

UNDERSTANDING THE TWO-BY-TWO TABLE

The authors agonized over whether this chapter should come so early in the book. Understanding the two-by-two table is difficult. You may never actually draw one again. The concepts inherent within the table are central to an understanding of prevalence and to an understanding of how prevalence can make a test valued by our specialist colleagues of little use in primary care. We suggest you read Chapters 2 and 3 as a unit.

The Perfect Screening Test

Imagine that a perfect test exists that is able to discriminate, with 100% accuracy, patients who have diabetes from those who do not (the "gold standard"), and that this new "perfect" test requires extensive use of tissue cultures, at a cost of $1000 per sample analyzed.

As part of a well-funded research project, you have found 1000 study subjects who carry a gene for diabetes. This gene causes 100% of the subjects to be diabetic and show abnormal serum glucose levels (7 to 15 mmol/L) on laboratory analysis. A second cohort of 1000 study subjects do not have the diabetes gene, do not have diabetes, and have serum glucose levels between 3 and 7 mmol/L.

Two-by-Two Table

Given the $1000 cost of this "perfect" test for diabetes, the realities of clinical practice dictate that we continue using the somewhat imperfect, but relatively inexpensive and easy-to-per-form 2-hour pc serum glucose test for routine diagnosis of diabetes. Many factors can influence the serum glucose level determined by 2-hour pc blood glucose test, such as foods consumed 1 to 2 days prior, or even 2 hours prior to the test, recent alcohol consumption, body weight, liver function, age, gender, and other variables.

Laboratory determination of the normal range for a 2-hour pc serum glucose is calculated by sampling thousands of 2-hour pc serum glucose tests from patients not considered to be diabetic, and then constructing a distribution curve from the results. The normal value for a 2-hour pc serum glucose is determined by identifying the serum glucose level in 95% of individuals whose serum glucose values fall under a bell curve (gaussian curve) (Figure 2–1). The 2.5% whose serum glucose is at either end of the bell curve are considered to have abnormal results.

Accuracy of the 2-hour pc serum glucose is determined by subjecting the 2000 people to the perfect test and to a 2-hour pc serum glucose test. Through 2-hour pc serum glucose testing of the 1000 diabetics confirmed by the perfect test, we learn that 100 have normal 2-hour pc serum glucose results. Thus, we have 900 true positives (labeled group A) and 100 false negatives (labeled group C). Similarly, there are 100 individuals with a high result on the 2-hour pc serum glucose test who by the perfect test are not diabetic. Thus, we have 100 false positives (labeled group B) and 900 true negatives (labeled group D).

When constructing a two-by-two table, each of the four boxes is always labeled the same: true positive(A) false positive(B), or false negative(C) true negative(D). A sample two-by-two table can easily be constructed using our artificial estimates and by following the "rules" of the two-by-two table, as explained and demonstrated in Figure 2–2. One simple way to use the two-by-two table is to total the contents of each of the four boxes outside of the two-by-two square (e.g., if the outside box totals are known, then simple addition or subtraction will give you the numbers missing from the other boxes).

When reading any article that uses the terms false positive, positive predictive value, negative predictive value, sensitivity, or specificity, it is essential that the article reports numbers which enable you to construct a two-by-two table. If the information provided is not sufficient to construct a two-by-two table, then the paper is not adequately transparent in providing important information and should be considered suspect.

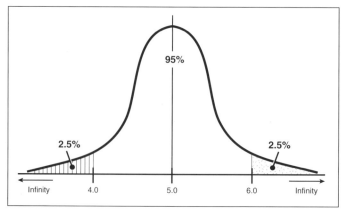

Figure 2–1   Distribution of 2–hr pc blood sugar results using a gaussian distribution. Normal values are those that fall between 2.5% of the lowest and 2.5% of the highest blood sugar values.

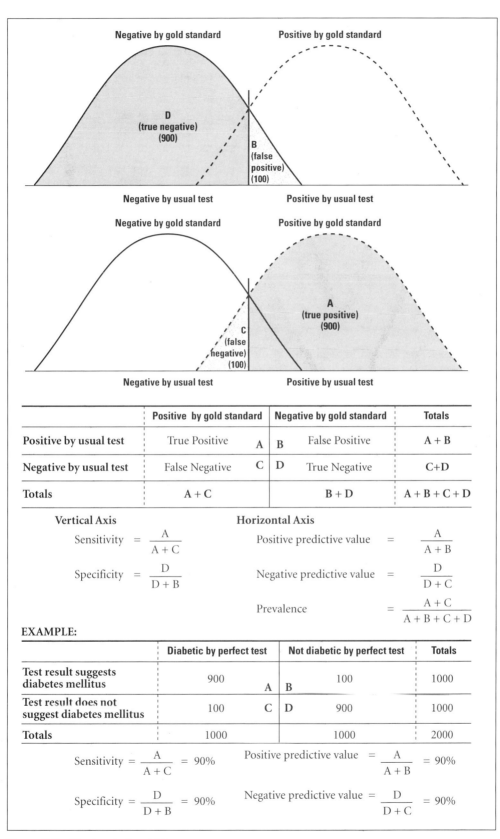

	Positive by gold standard		Negative by gold standard		Totals
Positive by usual test	True Positive	**A**	**B**	False Positive	**A + B**
Negative by usual test	False Negative	**C**	**D**	True Negative	**C+D**
Totals	**A + C**			**B + D**	**A + B + C + D**

Vertical Axis	Horizontal Axis
Sensitivity $= \dfrac{A}{A + C}$	Positive predictive value $= \dfrac{A}{A + B}$
Specificity $= \dfrac{D}{D + B}$	Negative predictive value $= \dfrac{D}{D + C}$
	Prevalence $= \dfrac{A + C}{A + B + C + D}$

EXAMPLE:

	Diabetic by perfect test		Not diabetic by perfect test		Totals
Test result suggests diabetes mellitus	900	**A**	**B**	100	1000
Test result does not suggest diabetes mellitus	100	**C**	**D**	900	1000
Totals	1000			1000	2000

$$\text{Sensitivity} = \frac{A}{A + C} = 90\% \qquad \text{Positive predictive value} = \frac{A}{A + B} = 90\%$$

$$\text{Specificity} = \frac{D}{D + B} = 90\% \qquad \text{Negative predictive value} = \frac{D}{D + C} = 90\%$$

Figure 2–2   The two-by two table.

Sensitivity

Sensitivity is defined as the ability of a diagnostic test to detect the presence of disease. How good is the 2-hour pc serum glucose test at detecting diabetes? Stated another way, how much confidence can you have that the patient does have diabetes when a "positive" result is reported from a 2-hour pc serum glucose test?

Comparing the results of our perfect test with the 2-hour pc serum glucose test, we know that 100 subjects known to have diabetes had a normal 2-hour pc serum glucose result. The calculation for sensitivity (ability of the 2-hour pc serum glucose test to detect those who have diabetes) is:

$$A / (A + C)$$

where A is the number of people shown to have diabetes by both tests, and C is the number of persons with a false negative result on the 2-hour pc serum glucose test. Therefore, the sensitivity is 900/(900+100), or 90%, which means that nine out of ten 2-hour pc serum glucose tests will accurately detect diabetes (see Figure 2–2).

Specificity

Specificity is defined as the ability of a test to detect the absence of disease. When a 2-hour pc serum glucose is reported as normal, how much confidence can you have that the patient does not have diabetes? When discussing this result with the patient, it is important to know what level of confidence can be had in making such a statement. The calculation of specificity is:

$$D / (D + B)$$

where D is the number of people with a normal result as determined by both tests, and B is the number of people in the false positive group (abnormal serum glucose level but confirmed by perfect test as not diabetic). Therefore, the specificity of the 2-hour pc serum glucose test is 900/(900+100), or 90%, which means that nine out of 10 of these patients are not diabetic, but 1 in 10 is diabetic, despite the normal result on the 2-hour pc serum glucose test (see Figure 2–2).

Positive Predictive Value (PPV)

The PPV is defined as the proportion of people undergoing the test, in whom we are confident the diagnosis of diabetes is correct. Using the 2-hour pc serum glucose and the perfect test, this proportion is calculated using the formula:

$$A / (A + B)$$

where A is again equal to the number of people in the true positive group, and B is the number of people in the false positive group. This means that the PPV will be strongly affected by the prevalence of disease. Using the numbers on the Table in Figure 2–2, the positive predictive value is 900/(900+100), and equals 90%. This can be interpreted as having confidence that 90% of the persons obtaining a 2-hour pc serum glucose result greater than 7.0 mmol/L are indeed diabetic (see Figure 2–2).

Negative Predictive Value (NPV)

The negative predictive value determines what the chance of finding a negative result is, and is calculated by the formula:

$$D / (D + C)$$

which is simply the true negatives divided by the total number who are reported normal, or 900/(900+100), providing a 90% negative predictive value.

In primary care, the true negative, D, is almost always high because of the low prevalence of disease in community-based populations which means that the NPV will always be high and hence of little value.

ASSESSING THE QUALITY OF ARTICLES DESCRIBING A NEW DIAGNOSTIC TEST

With a clear understanding of the two-by-two table, any study that evaluates a diagnostic test may be critically assessed. There are several questions that must be answered in the assessment process.

Does the study involve a POEM or a DOE?

Through the steps described in Chapter 1, you have decided to read a paper discussing a new diagnostic test. It may be useful to determine whether the test is a POEM (patient-oriented evidence that matters) or a DOE (disease-oriented evidence), before continuing with the paper. The pertinent questions are "What will the patient outcome be if the test result is positive?" and "Will the test detect a problem for which there is an effective and acceptable (to this individual) intervention that will alter the natural history of the disease in a positive way?"

Is the "gold standard" reasonable?

Any evaluation of a result must include an assessment of the sensitivity and specificity of a test. A gold standard, or "ideal" is required to construct a two-by-two table. Gold standards are non-existent, as are tests like the "perfect" test for diabetes. Therefore, the reader must make a judgment regarding the appropriateness of the gold standard used; if the gold standard used is too imperfect or not reasonable for judging the test, then there is little value in reading further. Many practitioners consider a throat swab to be the gold standard for detecting streptococcal infections of the throat; however, studies demonstrate that four physical signs, fever greater than 38.5°C, tender cervical lymph nodes, white pharyngeal exudate, and palatine stippling, have an 88% positive predictive value for *Streptococcus*, compared to a 75% PPV for the throat swab. The latex office strep test has a 93% PPV, and therefore may be considered the gold standard, with physical signs a close second.

Was blinding appropriate and adequately described?

Every study should be designed to reduce the risk of bias influencing the results. Numerous strategies for reducing bias will be discussed throughout this book. One of the fundamental strategies for reducing bias in studies is "blinding." If an individual is recording or interpreting results of a test, he or she must not know whether the test subject was part of the intervention group or the control group. Also, there must be several judges interpreting the results, and they must be blind to which study group the subject belongs, and to the interpretations of their colleagues. For example, a radiologist interpreting chest films in a study to evaluate a pneumonia therapy must be blind to which study group the patients belong.

Double-blinding

Double-blinding is commonly used in drug trials to reduce bias, and involves keeping those conducting the study blind as to which group subjects are in, and also keeping the subjects unaware of which study group they are in. An example of a double-blind trial is the so-called "N of One Trial".[1] If a patient has taken a single dose of a sleeping pill for the past five years, neither you nor the patient can know if the drug continues to help with sleep. A friendly pharmacist is willing to help determine the drug's effectiveness in this patient by matching the pill your patient is taking with an equal quantity of identical placebo. With the patient's understanding and consent, the pharmacist provides the patient with four bottles of medication; two containing seven pills each of active drug, and two containing seven pills each of placebo. The pharmacist has numbered all four bottles and has recorded which bottles contain the active drug or placebo. The physician and the patient are blind to which pills are in which bottle. All four bottles are given to the patient with instructions to keep a sleep diary for four weeks, taking pills from one bottle each week. On completion of the study, the pharmacist matches the active drug and placebo to the patient's sleep diary, thereby answering the question about the value of the drug for this patient. Since neither the physician nor the patient were able to differentiate the active drug from the placebo during the four week trial period, this is an example of both a double-blind trial and an N of One trial.

Are the study setting and study population comparable to your practice setting and population?

When assessing a study it is important to determine whether the study population roughly corresponds to the age and/or sex distribution, and other significant variables that comprise your practice population. Often, studies are conducted in tertiary care centers on highly selected patient populations that are significantly different from the typical practice populations. The conclusions of a study are suspect if the population is highly selected, and yet these conclusions are often extrapolated to everyone.

An important characteristic of a diagnostic test, particularly for family practitioners, is the test's ability to discriminate patients who do have the disease from patients who do not, despite the presence of similar symptoms. Ideally, the test would discriminate between those with similar symptoms early in the natural history of the disease. If a diagnostic test is only evaluated in people who clearly have or do not have the disease, then the test does not have the level of discriminatory power that is of practical value in your work.

The positive predictive value of a test is also influenced by the prevalence of the disease in the study population (see Chapter 3). A highly selected or filtered population, as seen in specialty referral practice, will have a different positive predictive value for a specific diagnostic test than in general and family practice where the prevalence of the disease will be lower. Most research studies assessing laboratory tests are conducted in selected or filtered populations, and these results should be applied to your practice with caution.

Is there adequate evaluation of the test to demonstrate reproducible results?

When assessing the value of a diagnostic test, a description of the results obtained by different individuals, using different study populations, and in different settings should be included. This description should be very "transparent," which means that based on the description of the methods provided, the study could be conducted again and obtain the same or similar results. If in conducting the study some interobserver variation was found, some discussion of, and explanation for, the findings should be part of the study report. The results of a study gain credibility if they are reproducible.

Does the definition of "normal" for this test make clinical sense?

Studies of diagnostic tests should include a definition of the normal value range for the test, and this definition must make clinical sense. Defining normal as two standard deviations from the mean does not always make clinical sense. For example, the use of a gaussian distribution (bell curve) to arrive at a definition of normal is inadvisable, as it does not usually fit with clinical reality (Figure 2–1). The tail of the bell curve goes to infinity, implying that a serum

TEACHING / LEARNING TIPS

- Query with students the sensitivity and specificity of tests they are using in the clinical setting by phoning the laboratory and asking the question.

- Examine an automated test report with test results that were not requested. There is a 5% chance that a normal test result is reported as abnormal.

- Using a peer-reviewed journal, ask students to check the calculations on assessment of a new test by constructing two-by-two tables directly from articles.

- Provide a group discussion about the concepts of the two-by-two table after everyone has read the basic material.

- Ask students to define the key terms that have been used.

- Using a clinical situation, take the available data and construct a two-by-two table. Calculate specificity, sensitivity, and positive and negative predictive values.

glucose level of 20, 40, 100, 500, or even 1000 mmol/L could possibly occur on testing; a situation that is clinically impossible as it would be incompatible with life. When the values that fall between the top and bottom 2.5% of a bell curve are used to define normal, the assumption is that all test results follow homogeneous distribution. This is usually not the case.

Another strategy for defining normal is to describe all results below the 95th percentile as normal. This strategy assumes that in the population being tested all diseases have the same prevalence. An extension of this assumption could be interpreted as the more tests a patient undergoes, the greater the likelihood of an abnormal result being reported. If a patient has two different tests, the chance of one abnormal result occurring is $.95 \times .95 = .90$. Extending this example out to twenty tests means a 1 in 3 chance exists that result will be incorrectly reported as abnormal.

A more sensible approach to determining a clinical definition of normal is to assess the ability of a diagnostic test to predict clinical events or outcomes. An example of this might be an attempt to statistically determine at what serum glucose level patients have an increased five-year mortality rate. This strategy is attractive, but the variability of individual outcomes and the sample size required to create statistically significant results make this approach impractical for studies of many diseases.

Fortunately, there are two practical and sensible methods to establish normal values. The diagnostic definition of normal identifies a range of diagnostic test results beyond which the probability of the presence of a disease is known. The probability of the presence of a disease is drawn from our discussion of the two-by-two table using the positive predictive value of a diagnostic test to establish the probability of disease being present.

The other approach to defining normal is the therapeutic definition. This approach sets the upper limit of normal as the level after which therapeutic interventions have been shown to do more good than harm. For example, in a 75-year-old female with a diastolic blood pressure of 90 mm Hg, the use of diuretics to reduce the blood pressure to 85 mm Hg may produce undesirable, or possibly risk-generating side effects. There are currently no studies demonstrating any benefit produced by lowering diastolic blood pressure below 90 mm Hg.[2] We do know that there is benefit in lowering blood pressure from 105 to 90 mm Hg. This knowledge allows us to set the upper limit for diastolic blood pressure in this individual at 95 or 100 mm Hg.

Does the test fit into a reasonable cluster of tests, and is the proposed sequence of testing reasonable?

Diagnostic tests should be conducted in a sequence. The first test should accurately measure the common symptoms that first appear in persons who have the disease. This same test may not be discriminatory enough to measure the second and third most common diseases. If the first test in the sequence produces a normal result, then the second test logically follows since it is more likely to detect the second most common disease causing these symptoms. Thus, if a study is reporting on a single diagnostic test, a description of how the test should be sequenced or clustered with other diagnostic tests in order to optimize the diagnostic efficiency should be included in the report.

QUESTIONS FOR EVALUATING STUDIES OF DIAGNOSTIC TESTS

1. Does the study involve a POEM or a DOE?
2. Is the gold standard reasonable?
3. Was blinding appropriate and adequately described?
4. Were the study setting and the study population appropriate for your practice?
5. Was there adequate evaluation of the test to demonstrate that the test was reproducible?
6. Was the normal for this test defined in an acceptable way?
7. Did the test fit into a reasonable cluster of tests, and was the sequence of testing proposed reasonable?

SUGGESTED ARTICLES TO EVALUATE

Catalona W, Smith D, Ratlif T, Dodds K, et al. Measurement of prostate-specific antigen in serum as a screening test for prostate cancer. N Engl J Med 1991;324:1156–1161.

Ewigman BG, Crane SP, Whitfeild CR, et al. Effects of prenatal ultrasound screening on perinatal outcomes. RADIUS study group. N Engl J Med 1993;329:821–827.

RECOMMENDED READING

Department of Clinical Epidemiology and Biostatistics, McMaster University Health Science Centre. How to read clinical journals. II: To learn about a diagnostic test. Can Med Assoc J 1981;124:703–710.

Jaescke R, Guyatt G, Sackett D. Users' guide to the medical literature. 3. How to use an article about a diagnostic test. A) Are the results of the study valid? JAMA 1994;271:389–391.

Jaescke R, Guyatt G, Sackett D. Users' guide to the medical literature. 3. How to use an article about a diagnostic test. B) What are the results and will they help me in caring for my patient? JAMA 1994;271: 703–707.

Sackett D, Haynes RB, Tugwell P. Clinical epidemiology: a basic science for clinical medicine. Toronto, Boston: Little Brown, 1985;p59.

REFERENCES

1.   Guyatt G, Sackett D, Taylor DW, Chong J, Roberts R, Pugsly S. Determining optimal therapy. Randomized trials on individual patients. New Engl J Med 1986;314:889–892.

2.   SHEP Co-operative Research Group. Prevention of stroke by antihypertensive drug treatment in older persons with isolated systolic hypertension. JAMA 1991;265:3255–3264.

CHAPTER 3

How Prevalence of Disease in a Practice Influences the Value of Tests

*The impact of disease prevalence in a population on the predictive value
of a test is a common source of misunderstanding about the differences in the
usefulness of tests in family and general practices compared to referral practice.*
Anonymous

The impact of disease prevalence on the value of diagnostic tests, especially screening tests, has led to fundamental misunderstandings between family and general practitioners and specialists regarding the usefulness of such tests. The way in which the prevalence of a disease influences the positive predictive value of a test is, mathematically, a relatively straightforward concept given an understanding of the two-by-two table. Through discussion and examples, this chapter addresses the source of these misunderstandings about the usefulness of medical tests.

LEARNING OBJECTIVES

Upon completion of this chapter the reader should be able to

1. understand how prevalence differences in varying populations change the value of diagnostic and screening tests;
2. better understand the source of controversy regarding the use of screening tests;
3. estimate the prevalence of common problems in clinical practice and determine the accuracy of this estimate;
4. determine the positive predictive value of several diagnostic tests used in clinical practice; and
5. use knowledge of the two-by-two table and prevalence to discuss with patients the relevance of tests to their needs.

THE IMPORTANCE OF PREVALENCE

Disease prevalence is an important issue for family and general practitioners to consider in clinical practice. A diagram created by Kerr White in the 1960s (Figure 3–1) illustrates that in a population of 1000 people during a one-month time period, only 25% experienced no illness, 50% experienced some illness but did not see their health care provider, 24% received health care from their usual provider, 1% were referred to a second physician or admitted to a nonteaching hospital, and fewer than 0.1% received care from a tertiary care center (teaching hospital).[1]

Almost all medical education and most research on diagnostic tests take place in teaching hospitals. Specialist researchers often extrapolate their experience, based on dealing with highly selected referral populations, to family and general practice, disregarding the difference in the prevalence of medical problems between the two settings. A perspective about the prevalence of health problems which has been developed in a teaching hospital is not relevant to primary care. A lack of understanding of this issue, combined with a modicum of arrogance that teaching hospitals are the centers of all "truth" in medicine, provides the basis for recurrent and fundamental misunderstandings about the value of tests and investigations in family and general practice.

The Study Population

One of the principles of evidence-based interpretation of study results is that the population used must be comparable to one's own clinical practice population. Every study must provide an accurate description of the sources and characteristics of the population included in the study. The absence of this basic demographic information makes the relevance of the recommendations in the study questionable. Adequate information will allow clinicians to decide if the conclusions of a study can be adjusted for application in their practices.

To make informed decisions about the applicability of study results to clinical practice, it is necessary to know the age and sex distribution of the individual practice population. Table 3-1 lists the prevalence of the 12 most common problems in the urban area of Hamilton-Wentworth, which has a population of approximately 500,000. Table 3–2 is taken from the same illness prevalence survey instrument but illustrates the prevalence for the Province of Ontario, which has a population of 10,000,000. The effect of age and sex on the prevalence of injuries from accidents across the Province of Ontario is demonstrated in Table 3–3. Table 3–4 lists the frequency with which the 15 most common problems are seen in five samples of North American family and general practices. Only the six most common problems represent more than 1% of the work load of primary care physicians. Table 3–5 allows comparison of the work load of primary care physicians in North America with the work load of primary care clinics that serve a poor and underhoused population in Curitiba, Brazil. Despite the difference in living conditions and economic status, the work loads are similar. Regional or local data on the prevalence of disease in a specific community may be difficult to find, but if available, comparisons can be made between the number of patients in a practice population with a specific diagnosis and the number expected based on community prevalence data.

An interesting exercise is to test the estimate of how many people in a practice should have a particular diagnosis and how many are actually identified. It can also be challenging to

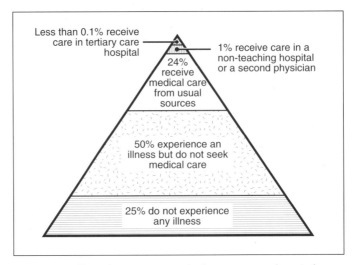

Figure 3–1 Illness in 1000 persons during a one-month period. Adapted from White et al. 1961.

attempt to explain a significant difference between the number of patients estimated to have a problem and the number known to have the diagnosis. For example, from the age and sex distributions of a practice population, one can estimate that there are 100 men between the ages of 60 and 75 years. The prevalence of angina pectoris in this population is approximately 15%, suggesting that 10 to 20 men in a practice should have this problem. On reviewing patient records, you find there are 32 recorded cases of angina pectoris. Is there a demographic explanation for its higher prevalence, or is angina pectoris being overdiagnosed? If the rate of smoking in your community is twice the provincial/state or national average, then it would not be surprising to find a higher prevalence of angina. This type of exercise can help practitioners better understand their practices, provide them with information that will help determine preventive priorities, and assist in assessing the value of specific diagnostic tests for their patients.

The Impact of the Prevalence of Disease

Sensitivity and specificity are on the vertical axis of the two-by-two table. As long as the percentage of false negatives (C) and false positives (B) of a test remains the same, the prevalence of a diagnosis does not affect the sensitivity or specificity of a test (Figure 3–2).

When we shift to the horizontal axis to calculate positive and negative predictive values, the prevalence of the disease has an impact. Figure 3–2 illustrates this impact where the prevalence is 2% (i.e., there are 40 diabetics and 1960 nondiabetics), 10% (i.e., 200 diabetics and 1800 nondiabetics), and 32% (i.e., 640 diabetics and 1360 nondiabetics). For all scenarios we are arbitrarily assuming 10% false positive and 10% false negative rates for the 2-hour pc serum glucose.

In populations where the prevalence of a condition is low (almost all diagnoses in family practice), the negative predictive value of a test is likely to be greater than 90%, which makes

Table 3–1   Prevalence of Illness during 1995 in Hamilton-Wentworth Region (500,000)*

Condition	Male %	Female %	Total %
1. Muscle and joint pain	13	21	17
2. Seasonal hay fever	15	15	15
3. Low back pain	12	11	11
4. High blood pressure	7	10	9
5. Allergies to foods, drugs	8	11	9
6. Respiratory problems	7	8	7
7. Cardiac problems	7	6	6
8. Gastrointestinal problems	6	6	6
9. Problems with vision	3	3	3
10. Diabetes	2	2	2
11. Thyroid problems	< 1	< 1	< 1
12. Cancer	< 1	< 1	< 1

*Data courtesy the Hamilton-Wentworth Department of Public Health

calculating the negative predictive value of little help in clinical decision making. This is why negative predictive values are rarely discussed in test evaluation.

The point illustrated by Kerr White, and the fact that almost all clinical research is carried out on highly filtered populations visiting major teaching hospitals, make it unlikely that many study results can be useful in family and general practice. Subsequent examples illustrate the importance of this concept, especially when a screening test for the entire population is being promoted by those who do their research in a tertiary care hospital.

Prevalence as a Source of Controversy

The prevalence of prostate cancer in 65-year-old men referred to a urology clinic at most teaching hospitals is approximately 70%, although prevalence in men under 70 years in a family and general practice is probably less than 10%. Urologists involved in research promote the benefits of annual screening using a prostate specific antigen (PSA) test for all men over age 50. Researchers argue that the test has excellent specificity (> 90%) and sensitivity for early detection of carcinoma of the prostate. However, after confirmation of prostate cancer by biopsy, the positive predictive value for PSA testing was found to range from 8 to 33%. These findings suggest that at best, 67% of men, and at worst, 92%, will have an unnecessary biopsy and face the associated risk of bleeding and other complications.[2] Guidelines from urology associations state that every man over the age of 50 should have an annual screening PSA test. Urologists argue that general physicians and epidemiologists opposed to this recommendation are misguided, since early detection of cancer is clearly the right thing to do.[3] Consider the PPPP example for patients on page 137 to illustrate further the prevalence issue and how it provides a source of controversy between primary care physicians and subspecialists.

The evidence-based approach to family and general practice cannot endorse the urologists' guidelines or recommendations for several reasons. The first reason relates directly to the

Table 3–2   Prevalence of Illness in the Province of Ontario in 1994 (10,000,000)*

Condition	Male %	Female %	Total %
1. Seasonal hay fever	15	18	17
2. Pain in joints or muscle	11	16	14
3. Allergies to foods, drugs	7	9	8
4. High blood pressure	7	8	8
5. Low back pain	7	7	7
6. Respiratory problems	6	6	6
7. Gastrointestinal problems	5	5	5
8. Cardiac problems	5	5	5
9. Problems with eyes	2	3	3
10. Diabetes	2	2	2
11. Thyroid problems	1	4	2
12. Cancer	1	2	2

*Data courtesy the Hamilton-Wentworth Department of Public Health

Table 3–3   Injuries from Accidents during 1994 by Age Groups: Prevalence in the Province of Ontario*

Age (years)	Male	Female
1. 0–11	7%	6%
2. 12–19	18%	11%
3. 20–44	16%	9%
4. 45–64	10%	7%
5. 65+	5%	7%

* Data provided courtesy the Ontario Ministry of Health

issue of prevalence; the prevalence of prostate cancer in 50-year-old men is less than 1%, meaning that before one true positive PSA is found, 200 men will have to be tested.

The low prevalence of prostate cancer in family and general practice means that 67 to 92% of positive PSA tests are actually false positive. These men will undergo repeated blood tests and biopsy for reassurance that they were false positive. The anxiety the patient experiences as a result of a test result indicating he may have cancer is immeasurable; once a patient has been asked to undergo repeat PSA testing our ability to reassure him diminishes rapidly. Convinc-

Table 3–4   Problems Recorded as the Most Common Reasons for Visits to Family Physicians in Five Surveys of Canadian and American Practices[9]

Condition (ICHPPC Classification)	Percentage of Visits
1. Uncomplicated hypertension	11
2. Rhinitis (allergic or other)	9
3. Pharyngitis (including URI)	7
4. Anxiety disorders	3
5. Depression	2
6. Preventive health procedures	2
7. Contraceptive advice	1
8. Acute or chronic cough	1
9. Well-baby check	1
10. Nutritional advice (obesity)	> 1
11. Diabetes mellitus	> 1
12. Abdominal pain	> 1
13. Otitis media	> 1
14. Lower urinary tract infection	> 1
15. Heart failure	> 1

Table 3–5   The Sixteen Most Common Reasons for Visits to Family Health Clinics in Curitiba, Brazil (Serving Favilas or Poor Areas)*

1. Upper respiratory infections	9. Asthma/bronchitis
2. Hypertension	10. Headache
3. Well baby/child care	11. Low back pain
4. Diarrhea	12. Vaginitis
5. Abdominal pain	13. Prenatal care
6. Dermatitis	14. Parasitic infection
7. Pharyngitis	15. Otitis media
8. Anxiety	16. Pap. smear

*Data courtesy the Secretary of Health, City of Curibita, 1995

ing the patient that he is well after further tests are negative, given that no one can provide 100% assurance of the absence of disease, adds a further challenge to a very difficult situation. To date, we do not have clear evidence of the specificity or sensitivity of PSA testing.

The lower the prevalence of any problem in the population, the more tests are necessary to detect the true positive. What appear to be only minor weaknesses in a test (2 to 4% false positive rates), are exaggerated when repeated hundreds or thousands of times to detect a true positive (i.e., the false positives generated overwhelm the benefits of detecting the rare true positive). The lower the disease prevalence in a population, the more important the false positive and false negative rates attributed to the test become.

The second reason for the evidence-based practitioner's opposition to mass PSA testing is that the natural history of prostate cancer is not clearly understood. Eighty to 85% of men die *with* the disease and not *from* it. Prostate cancer progresses and metastasizes slowly; the disease usually goes undetected and most men die of other causes. The 15 to 20% of men who have a more aggressive disease fall into two groups: those with moderately aggressive disease who become symptomatic from the disease or the metastases, and those with very aggressive disease who rapidly deteriorate and die within months or a year after diagnosis. Men suffering from the most aggressive disease tend to be young and do not to respond to any therapy. The

Prevalence of diabetes	Sensitivity	Specificity	Positive predictive value	Negative predictive value
Normal population 2%	91%	91%	17%	99%
Obese elderly population 10%	91%	91%	53%	99%
Cree 32%	91%	91%	83%	96%
Axis	Vertical	Vertical	Horizontal	Horizontal

Figure 3–2   The impact of disease prevalence.

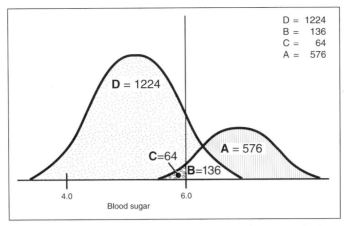

Figure 3–3   A 32% prevalence of diabetes in Northern Ontario Cree Indians.

men with the moderately aggressive disease, who represent approximately 8 to 12% of prostate cancer patients, appear to respond to some therapies, including radical prostatectomy. This latter procedure, however, carries with it several risks which include mortality (1–3%); complete incontinence (7%); any incontinence (27%); and impotence (32%).[4]

Unfortunately, the PSA test (or any other test) cannot discriminate between the three groups of men with different natural histories of the disease, nor is there any way of determining which individual will suffer which course. Screening all men over the age of 50 will result in large numbers of false positives. Once those that are true positives for cancer of the prostate have been confirmed, 80 to 85% will undergo radical treatment. Three percent of men with confirmed prostate cancer will die from the disease or treatment, and one-third will have a diminished quality of life in the absence of any benefit. Eight to 12% of men may benefit from early detection and treatment, but for those with more aggressive disease, no intervention appears to alter their rapid disease progression. The PSA, which is useful to urologists in monitoring prostate cancer, should not be used as a screening test in family and general practice as it has the potential to do more harm than good.

From this example, the way in which the prevalence of a disease causes misunderstanding and conflict between academic specialists producing clinical guidelines and family and general practitioners is demonstrated.

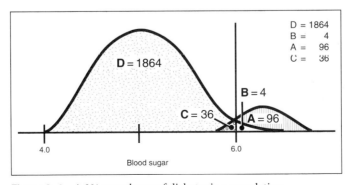

Figure 3–4   A 2% prevalence of diabetes in a population.

THE IMPACT OF WATCHFUL WAITING

The concept of "watchful waiting" is particularly important to family and general practitioners. Starfield estimates that 40% of patients presenting with new problems in family and general practice get better without a specific diagnosis ever being established.[5] A strategy used by family and general practitioners is to monitor individuals presenting with nonspecific signs or symptoms for several weeks. As the signs and symptoms early in the evolution of a disease become more specific, a hypothesis about the diagnosis may emerge. During this period of "watchful waiting" the pretest likelihood (see definition in glossary) of the problem being a disease for which there is a diagnostic test will increase. By waiting until there is a greater pretest likelihood of the disease being present, the prevalence of the disease in this observed "population" rises, and the risk of a false positive or a false negative test result is reduced. The concept of improving the pretest likelihood is illustrated in Figure 3–5. If a test with a 95% specificity is carried out on a patient with a 40% pretest likelihood of having the disease, and the test result is positive, then there is a > 90% chance of a true positive result. However, if the pretest likelihood is less than 10% (common in general and family practice), the test result loses its value, with a < 40% chance of the results being a true positive. If the specificity of the test drops from 95 to 75%, then the 40% pretest likelihood results in a 60% chance of the test result being a true positive. Thus, Figure 3–5 provides a visual image of the relationship between the pretest likelihood of a patient having a disease and the specificity of the test. This knowledge should help determine whether a test will offer greater diagnostic benefit than clinical judgment. The so-called "tincture of time" plays an important role in improving the positive predictive value of a diagnostic test.[6]

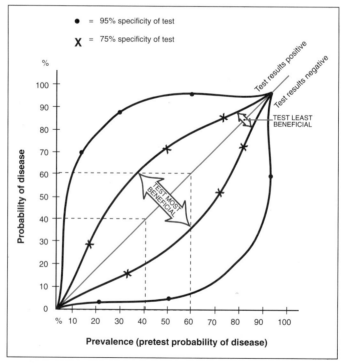

Figure 3–5   The impact of prevalence of disease in a population on the pretest likelihood.

TEACHING / LEARNING TIPS

- Have students determine the prevalence of common disorders in clinical practice and compare those with Table 3–2.

- Have students draw a two-by-two table (as shown in Figure 2–2) and do the calculations for a population of 2000 where the prevalence was 2% or 33%.

- Ask students to participate in two or three exercises where they estimate the pretest likelihood of a diagnosis using knowledge of prevalence of the condition. Discuss the value of doing the test in assisting them in making a diagnosis. Is the test better than clinical judgment?

- Lead a discussion on the impact of prevalence on guidelines produced in a tertiary care center for use in a primary care center.

- Provide students with reading on subjects where guidelines produced in a tertiary care setting are not helpful in a primary care setting because of the prevalence of the disease in family and general practice.

- Lead a discussion on the theories of diagnostic decision making. How do these theories assist in making diagnostic tests more useful?

- Whenever a student proposes to conduct a diagnostic test, ask why, ask for a prevalence estimate for the hypothesized diagnosis, and the pretest likelihood of the disease.

- Use the Physician-Patient Partnership Paper to assist a patient who wants a PSA test (see page 137).

When first seeing a patient, the primary care physician estimates the severity of the problem, usually from the patient's appearance (especially if the patient is well known to the physician), and then begins gathering information that helps to formulate a diagnosis. The ongoing debate about the diagnostic decision-making process in clinical medicine has resulted in the formulation of several theories to explain the process of diagnostic reasoning in physicians. One theory proposes that a physician cannot deal with every possible diagnosis when seeing each patient, so he/she formulates one or two hypotheses within a few seconds of observing the patient and then works toward ruling these hypotheses out. Another theory proposes that in the first few minutes of a patient encounter the physician is reminded of a similar patient with a specific diagnosis and begins to analyze how this patient's signs and symptoms correspond with those of the previous patient.[7,8] These are very superficial explanations of complex theories; further details can be found by consulting the references. Generally, previous knowledge and experience play a major role. Furthermore, if physicians practice in a patient-centered way, the fears, perceptions, and anxieties of the patient also play an important role in influencing their diagnostic thinking.

THE PRETEST LIKELIHOOD

The decision to order tests should be based on the pretest likelihood of detecting abnormality, which is based on your clinical judgment, coupled with the idea that the test will further contribute to confirming a diagnosis. A dramatic example of the importance of the pretest likelihood is found in the use of tests to diagnose the cause of chest pain. The likelihood of a 30-year-old man with chest wall pain having abnormal coronary arteries on an angiogram is low (estimated at about 5%). However, a 62-year-old man with signs and symptoms of angina pectoris has a very high pretest likelihood of having abnormal coronary arteries on a coronary arteriogram (estimated at 94%). How useful will an exercise ECG test be in helping in the decision-making process around each of these individuals? An exercise ECG test is relatively inexpensive and simple to administer, yet more importantly, it is noninvasive when compared to the gold standard provided by coronary arteriography. Unfortunately, the exercise ECG test is considerably less than perfect. A positive exercise ECG test in a 30-year-old male has a positive predictive value of only 26% An experienced clinician is unlikely to proceed to an invasive procedure such as a coronary arteriogram, with only 26% confidence in the patient having coronary heart disease. More confidence should be placed in the physician's own clinical judgment in this situation than anything contributed by the test. If we assess the 62-year-old man suffering from chest pain, a positive stress ECG test moves a 94% likelihood of coronary artery stenosis to 99%, which adds little to the clinician's own judgment.

In both cases, the prevalence of the disorder greatly influences the pretest likelihood of finding any abnormality in the coronary arteries. The use of this stress ECG test contributed little to determining whether more invasive and expensive arteriography should be conducted.

One might assume that the use of a stress ECG test to diagnose chest pain is useless. However, in some situations the pretest likelihood of coronary artery disease is less clear and the test may be helpful. For example, in a 45-year-old man with chest pain of suspected cardiac origin, the prevalence of coronary artery disease is 46%. The important question is whether to subject this man to an invasive procedure. If this man has a positive exercise ECG test, the positive predictive value for ischemic heart disease is estimated at 85%. In this scenario, the stress ECG plays a significant role in the clinical decision making.[9]

Prevalence figures should be readily available but are, in fact, hard to get. Once physicians realize how important prevalence is in interpreting the usefulness of a test they will perhaps begin to demand them.

QUESTIONS TO ASK WHEN REVIEWING ARTICLES DEALING WITH DISEASE PREVALENCE

1. Is the proposed test a POEM or a DOE?
2. Are the population characteristics adequately described?
3. Is adequate information provided to construct a two-by-two table?
4. How does the prevalence of the condition in the study population correspond to the prevalence in clinical practice? Does the difference eliminate the usefulness of results?
5. What is the natural history of the detected disease? Is there an intervention that alters the natural history of the disease?
6. Does the impact of the false positive or false negative rate estimated in one's practice outweigh any benefit that might arise from using the test?

SUGGESTED ARTICLES TO EVALUATE

Brawer MK, Chetner MP, Beatie J, et al. Screening for prostatic carcinoma with prostatic specific antigen. J Urol 1992;147:841–845.

Mandel JS, Bond JH, Church TR, et al. Reducing mortality from colorectal cancer by screening for fecal occult blood. N Eng J Med 1993;328:1365–1371.

RECOMMENDED READING

Jaeschke R, Guyatt G, Sackett D. Users' guide to the medical literature. III. How to use an article about a diagnostic test. B. What are the results and will they help me in caring for my patient? JAMA 1994; 271:703–707.

REFERENCES

1. White KL, Williams TF, Greenburg BG. The ecology of medical care. N Eng J Med 1961;265: 885–892.

2. Mettlin C, Lee F, Drago J, et al. The American Cancer Society National Prostate Cancer Detection Project: Findings of the detection of early prostate cancer in 2425 men. Cancer 1991;67:2949–2958.

3. The Canadian Task Force on the Periodic Health Examination. The Canadian guide to clinical preventive health care. Ottawa: Minister of Supply and Services, 1994;812–825.

4. Fleming C, Wasson JH, Albertsen PC, et al. A decision analysis of alternative treatment strategies for clinically localized prostate cancer. JAMA 1993;269:2650–2658.

5. Starfield B. Is primary care essential? Lancet 1994;344:1129–1133.

6. Rosser W. Approach to diagnosis by primary care clinicians and specialists: Is there a difference? J Fam Pract 1996;42:139–144.

7. Schmidt HG, Norman GR, Boshuizen HPA. Cognitive perspective on medical expertise: theory and implications. Acad Med 1990;65:611–621.

8. Elstein AS, Kagan N, Shulman IS, et al. Methods and theory in the study of medical inquiry. J Med Educ 1972;47:85–92.

9. Sackett DL, Haynes RB, Tugwell P. Clinical Epidemiology: A Basic Science for Clinical Medicine. Toronto: Little Brown, 1985.

CHAPTER 4

Advising Patients about Prognosis

———

Prognostics do not always prove prophecies—at least
the wisest prophets make sure of the event first.
Horace Walpole

When patients are told that they have a disease, they usually want to know its expected course. The more serious the illness, the more the patient wants to know about the "natural history" of the disease. The physician is put under pressure to predict outcome. This chapter discusses our ability to scientifically prognosticate about disease, given our ignorance of the natural history of many illnesses and our inability to predict how any one individual will respond to a threat to their well-being.

LEARNING OBJECTIVES

Upon completion of this chapter the reader should be able to

1. understand the importance of the natural history of a disease;
2. understand ways in which bias may have an impact on determining the prognosis of an illness; and
3. determine if an article about prognosis is relevant to the patient population in his/her practice.

Whenever a physician decides there is evidence to make a specific diagnosis, the patient's first questions usually are: What does this mean? How long will I live? How will the problem affect my lifestyle and quality of life? It is important that the physician provide the most thoughtful prognosis possible. For some patients, not knowing and imagining the worst can generate more anxiety than knowing they have a potentially fatal disease.

When attempting to predict the outcome for a well-known disease such as colon cancer, even the most experienced clinicians have been surprised by some patients who survive for years and others who decline quickly. Despite a sound knowledge of the natural history of a disease, the physician will find that individual physical and emotional responses to chronic or life-threatening disease can vary.

Knowledge of the natural history of an illness is often lacking, especially that of cancer. Further complicating this situation is the fact that patients typically present to their primary care clinician early in the course of illness when symptoms are nonspecific. Many of these non-specific problems resolve with little more than "watchful waiting" or a "tincture of time," the effect enhanced by a trusting physician-patient relationship and liberal reassurance. Although critics may call such strategies unscientific, there is a growing body of evidence that this behavior by family and general practitioners is cost effective. In countries where a high percentage of care is delivered by family and general practitioners rather than specialists, health care delivery is more cost effective.[1]

If a problem evolves to meet diagnostic criteria defined by the International Classification of Diseases (I.C.D.-10)*, or more relevant to family and general practitioners, the ICHPPC** classification system, and we know the natural history of the diagnosed disease, how do we use this knowledge?[2] The natural history of the most common human affliction, the cold or upper respiratory infection (URI), is well described. The PPPP for the URI found on p. 110 illustrates the importance of knowing the natural history of a disease to appropriately treat it.

Knowledge of the URI would help people understand that no intervention available today, including antibiotics, alters its natural history. This knowledge would allow individuals to better judge if their cold varied enough from the normal course of the illness to warrant medical attention. The appropriate use of this knowledge could adversely affect the multi-billion dollar over-the-counter pharmaceutical industry which depends on people believing that their remedies influence the natural history of the cold (see Chapter 15.3).

Study Biases

Examining studies on prognosis provides an opportunity to discuss the ways bias can enter a study. The Dictionary of Epidemiology defines bias as "any trend in the collection, analysis, interpretation, publication, or review of data that can lead to conclusions that are systematically different from the truth."[3] Bias occurs in many prognosis studies when a proper inception cohort is not assembled. By admitting patients to a study at the time of diagnosis or on arrival at a tertiary care clinic, the conclusions derived from the subsequent prospective study may be incorrect since this flawed procedure involves several types of bias. Studies whose inception cohorts were assembled at the time of arrival at a tertiary care center are commonly found in the literature.

Lead Time Bias

If the natural history of a disease is known and we wish to determine if a medical intervention can alter it, the point in the natural history at which measurement begins is important.

For example, a 10 mm in diameter breast mass detected by mammography is at a different point than a 2 to 10 cm mass detected manually by the patient (the way 90% of breast cancers are detected). The expectations for the outcome of these two situations are different, yet the starting point for intervention measurement is considered to be the time of diagnosis. As a result of early detection, the woman in the first example was found to have cancer of the breast 1 1/2 years after the disease "started." She lived 6 1/2 years. In the second example, cancer was detected only when the woman herself felt a 7 cm mass in her breast, 4 1/2 years after the onset of disease. She lived 3 1/2 years after diagnosis. Surgeons, oncologists, and radiologists will argue that early intervention added 3 years to the life of "A," when in fact there was no effect on the natural history of the disease. Both women lived for 8 years after the onset of the cancer. This phenomenon of apparent prolongation of life with early detection is known as lead time bias (Figure 4–1).

Any study dealing with the prognosis of disease should have a clearly defined inception cohort to ensure that the starting point for all patients is the same (e.g., all patients have a 10-mm lesion at biopsy initially detected by mammography, no evidence of metastasis, and

*I.C.D.-10 was produced by the World Health Organization (WHO) in 1994 and is the most widely used diagnostic classification system in the world.

**ICHPPC (International Classification of Health Problems in Primary Care), produced in 1992 for the WHO, is a classification system for family physicians based on "reason for encounter" and relates to I.C.D.-10.

no comorbid conditions such as another cancer or severe heart disease that might have an impact). Good studies on prognosis describe how the inception cohort was assembled and its characteristics.

Centripetal Bias

Centripetal bias occurs when a referral center has an outstanding reputation which draws people to it from outside its geographical location. An inception cohort assembled at the time of arrival at such a center will be affected by factors such as the patient's ability to afford to travel to this center and the diagnostic and management capabilities of the referral source. For example, if a large American center attracted women with breast cancer from around the world, only those who could pay travel and health care costs would be included in the study. The effects of poverty, nutrition, depression, and access to therapy could influence the natural history of breast cancer but would not be considered in the study. The centripetal bias created by the reputation and cost of treatment at the center means that studies conducted on its population will produce results that may not apply to your practice population.

Popularity Bias

Popularity bias may occur when people with specific diagnoses are treated differently than those with other conditions. This is most likely to happen in tertiary care centers with an international reputation for treatment of specific diseases where there is incentive to admit patients with such diagnoses. The preferential treatment may take the form of higher admission rates, longer stay, accelerated access to diagnostic tests, special attention for therapies, and extra attention given because of participation in clinical trials.

Referral Bias

The importance of referral bias to family physicians attempting to interpret the literature can not be overemphasized. Referral patterns in a community often do not follow predictable

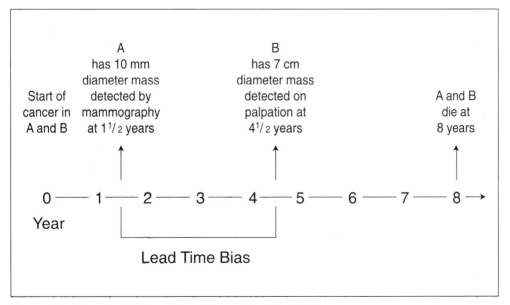

Figure 4–1 The natural history of breast cancer (lead time bias).

TEACHING / LEARNING TIPS

- Ask students to identify a patient with a chronic condition and review the literature on the prognosis. Use the medical literature to make points about natural history and prognosis.

- Evaluate students' knowledge of the definitions covered in this chapter.

- Conduct a tutorial on the natural history of disease. Ask students to list common cancers and other illnesses with known natural histories.

- Have students discuss how an unknown natural history influences the study of five-year survival rates in cancer.

- Review and evaluate the criteria used for determining five-year cancer survival rates.

- Choose any randomized controlled trial from a reputable journal and identify potential sources of bias in the study. Have they been appropriately dealt with?

patterns. In communities without tertiary care hospitals, physicians can refer patients to a number of centers. This makes a cohort group assembled at a referral clinic unlikely to provide a random or even a reasonable sample of the community's population, unless there is only one referral center serving the entire population.

Diagnostic Access Bias

Diagnostic access bias is the differing ability to access diagnostic facilities. If the starting point for assembling a cohort for a prospective study is a positive MRI, does every member of the population have equal access to the scanner? Many centers require consultations or special referrals from physicians, and patients may not be in a position to pay the costs or may require weeks or months to find the money.

Diagnostic Suspicion Bias

Blinding and double blinding are described in Chapter 2. If a clinician suspects a patient in a blinded trial belongs either to the placebo or intervention group, diagnostic suspicion bias may influence the physician's actions towards that patient.

Expectation Bias

An expectation bias is created by second-guessing what is happening in a trial or with a patient based on prior knowledge. Ideally, participants in a trial should know as little about the trial as is ethically permissible. Some studies intentionally withhold information, such as x-ray, ECGs, or pathology results, from the researchers who are interpreting the study results in order to reduce the expectation bias that would occur if they were aware of the diagnosis.

Some important outcomes can not be blinded. For example, a randomized controlled trial of episiotomy sought to show that episiotomy provides little benefit to most women, and that a midline episiotomy extending into a fourth degree tear has a worse outcome than a natural tear.[4] The study used standardized instruments and objective nonphysician personnel who assessed pain and discomfort in women who did or did not have an episiotomy. This approach reduced the bias, when the outcome could not be blinded. When reviewing any paper describing a clinical trial, blinding is an important issue; if blinding is not dealt with in a transparent way, the paper is weak and should be rejected. If the trial outcome cannot be blinded, as in the above example, evaluation of how the issue was addressed is necessary to determine whether the researcher's strategy is acceptable.

EXTRANEOUS FACTORS

When reviewing papers dealing with prognosis, it is important to be confident that extraneous factors that may have affected the prognosis have been appropriately addressed. In a study dealing with any advantage of total mastectomy over lumpectomy for breast cancer, one might hypothesize that tumor location may be important; a tumor adjacent to the axillary lymph nodes would likely metastasize more rapidly, resulting in a poorer prognosis. This would be considered an extraneous factor that should be dealt with in the analysis of the study. In all studies of prognosis any extraneous factors that might influence the prognosis should be identified and analyzed.

OUTCOMES

Once a proper cohort is assembled and followed carefully, the point of completion of the study, or endpoint, must be clearly defined. Death is the absolute outcome, but other endpoints include loss of independence, change in the quality of life, and an event specific to the disease (e.g., in a study following individuals suffering from angina pectoris, myocardial infarction may represent the appropriate endpoint). Whatever the endpoint, it must be clearly defined and described so the outcome of the study can be extrapolated to patients in an individual practice. If the description of the endpoint is not transparent, interpretation becomes difficult and the study results unclear.

QUESTIONS TO ASK WHEN REVIEWING ARTICLES ON PROGNOSIS

1. Is the study of prognosis dealing with a POEM or a DOE?
2. Was an appropriate inception cohort assembled? Was the description of the process transparent?
3. Was the pattern of referrals for assembly of the cohort described in a transparent fashion? Were potential biases in referrals identified and dealt with appropriately?
4. Were all those in the inception cohort accounted for at the end of the study?
5. Were the outcome criteria objective?
6. Was the outcome assessment conducted by individuals blind to the trial groups?
7. Was there an appropriate adjustment for extraneous factors in the assessment?
8. How will this study impact on your practice?

SUGGESTED ARTICLES TO EVALUATE

Fisher B, Bauer M, Margolese R, et al. Five-year results of a randomized controlled trial comparing total mastectomy and segmental mastectomy with or without radiation in the treatment of breast cancer. New Eng J Med 1985;312(11):665–681.

Meanwell CA, Kelly KA, Wilson S, et al. Young age as a prognostic factor in cervical cancer: Analysis of population based data from 10,022 cases. Br Med J 1988;296:386–391.

Miller AB, Baines CJ, To T, Wall C. Canadian National Breast Screening Study: 1. Breast cancer detection and death rates among women aged 40 to 49. Can Med Assoc J 1992;147:1459–1476.

RECOMMENDED READING

Laupacis A, Wells G, Richardson WS, Tugwell P. Users guide to the medical literature. How to use an article about prognosis. JAMA 1994;272:234–237.

Department of Clinical Epidemiology and Biostatistics, McMaster University. How to read clinical journals: III. To learn the clinical course and prognosis of disease. Can Med Assoc J 1981;124:869–872.

Sackett DL, Haynes RB, Tugwell P. Clinical Epidemiology: A Basic Science for Clinical Medicine. Toronto: Little Brown, 1984.

REFERENCES

1.   Starfield B. Is primary care essential? Lancet 1994;344:1129–1133.

2.   Lamberts H, Wood M. International Classification of Health Problems in Primary Care. Oxford: Oxford University Press, 1992.

3.   Last JM. A Dictionary of Epidemiology, Third Edition. New York: Oxford University Press, 1995:15.

4.   Klein MC, Gauthier RJ, Robbins JM, et al. Relationship of episiotomy to perineal trauma and morbidity, sexual dysfunction, and pelvic floor relaxation. Am J Obstet Gynecol 1994;171:591–598.

CHAPTER 5

How to be Confident About a Cause-and-Effect Relationship

We are too much accustomed to attribute to a single cause that which
is the product of several, and the majority of our controversies come from that.
Baron Justice von Liebig

Family and general practitioners are continually frustrated by reports in the media that consumption of or exposure to a specific food, drug, or airborne toxin results in a predictable, and usually negative, outcome. Does drinking six cups of coffee daily cause cancer? Does eating fish daily cause stomach cancer? Does using aluminum cooking pots cause Alzheimer's disease? Does eating beef from cows with "mad cow disease" cause mental deterioration? The purpose of this chapter is to help the physician review the articles that provide the basis for these claims to determine if a cause-and-effect relationship has been established.

Key terms introduced in this chapter are factor analysis, analysis of variance, relative risk, odds ratio, temporal relationship, and dose-response gradient. Consult the glossary for definitions.

LEARNING OBJECTIVES

Upon completion of this chapter the reader should be able to

1. critically review an article that proposes a cause-and-effect relationship;
2. determine if the proposed relationship is sound; and
3. determine if the cause-and-effect relationship has meaning for their patients and their health-related behavior.

ANALYZING CAUSE-AND-EFFECT RELATIONSHIPS

Over the past 25 years, software packages such as SPSS (Statistical Package for Social Sciences) have made it relatively easy for researchers to analyze data sets collected for administrative purposes. Any "relationship" detected by SPSS analysis on what some might call a "fishing expedition" could be the basis for a hypothesis about a cause-and-effect relationship. Making these revelations available to the media can be the route to international fame. These hypotheses, derived from retrospective analyses, feed the media's insatiable appetite for dramatic statements about fearful consequences. Inappropriate reporting can lead to widespread behavioral change that is not justified. A simple metaphor for factorial analysis or analysis of variance for hypothesis generation is that of duck hunting by lying flat on your back in a marsh, aiming a shotgun straight up in the air and firing blindly until something comes down. The desirable outcome of this style of analysis should be the generation of hypotheses leading to formal studies to establish a cause-and-effect relationship.

The Impact of Methodology on Cause-and-Effect Relationships

The most efficient way to analyze cause-and-effect claims is to critically assess the paper on which the claims are based. Knowledge of the strengths of different methodologies (see Chapter 1) is particularly important in analyzing articles making cause-and-effect relationship claims. A claim of causation often arises from the method known as the analysis of variance (ANOVA). This is the weakest methodology for determining causation because it does not control for any form of bias. Cohort studies are subject to considerable bias and case-control studies examining groups retrospectively are subject to even more bias.

A prospective randomized controlled trial (RCT) is the best way to establish a cause-and-effect relationship. An RCT conducted on a population that resembles a family and general practice should provide confidence in the strength of the relationship, especially if the trial has been replicated. However, a causal claim rarely arises from such trials as they are often impractical, especially to answer the types of cause-and-effect relationships in which the public shows the greatest interest.

From an ethics viewpoint, no one has ever done, or would do an RCT of persons randomized to smoke or not to smoke for a lifetime. However, there is such strong epidemiologic association from hundreds of studies—including studies involving an entire country and studies between many different groups and cultures—that the link between tobacco smoking and lung cancer is considered sound by everyone except cigarette manufacturers. This is an exceptional situation in which the epidemiologic evidence from many sources is so convincing that an RCT, or even a case-control trial, is unnecessary to prove the strength of the cause-and-effect relationship. The link between smoking and cancer, or smoking and respiratory disease is the most notable exception to the rule that cause-and-effect relationships usually require an RCT to be convincing.

The literature on which most of the widely publicized cause-and-effect relationships is based is often grounded in weak methodology; this reason alone should be comforting when advising patients that the links are speculative only, and that it is premature for them to change their behavior patterns. Unfortunately, emotion based on inadequate evidence of a relationship often rules the day, as illustrated by the "mad cow disease" scare emanating from the United Kingdom and affecting beef consumption around the world. It is difficult to understand the worldwide reaction to "mad cow disease" when thousands of people are dying from the tobacco-related diseases that continue to take their toll of human health.

Bias in Cause-and-Effect Studies

Articles must be critiqued on the basis that any inherent bias may lead to the wrong conclusions. For example, to determine whether jogging leads to a reduction in heart attack rates in middle-aged men, you would assemble a well-described group of middle-aged men and randomize them to one of two groups: one that jogs daily and one that does not. After following both groups for a minimum of 10 years, you could answer your question. Such a study would be extremely expensive and, because of dropouts, require such a large cohort that it would be impracticable. You could assemble a cohort of men who do and do not jog and follow them simultaneously for 10 or more years. The inherent methodologic problem here is that men who choose to jog are likely to have characteristics that place them at reduced risk of heart disease in the first place when compared to those who choose not to jog (e.g., weight differential, lifetime activity levels, type of work, socioeconomic level, education, level of life stress, smoking, etc.). A well-conducted cohort study may be convincing and may identify variables that influence causation, but the cohort study will always be weaker than an RCT because of the potential for uncontrolled bias.

The case-control study, which by definition is retrospective, presents even greater weakness. A case-control study assembles a group of men who have suffered one or more heart attacks and then compares them to a group of similar men that have not suffered any cardiovascular events. Using this method to identify a cause-and-effect linkage requires retrospective measurement of the daily exercise levels of the two groups. The number of potential biases in the two groups assembled in this way considerably exceeds those identified for cohort studies, providing even less support for cause-and-effect relationships (Table 5–1).

The fact that the Japanese have a 40% lower cardiovascular disease rate when compared to the general Canadian population presents a temptation to provide a dietary explanation for the difference, yet there are so many cultural variables between the two societies that could influence the incidence of cardiovascular disease that it is meaningless to draw any conclusions. One recently detected variable in the cause of cardiovascular disease is hypothesized to be a sense of security and control over one's destiny. The influence of this characteristic may be strengthened in Japanese society because of its homogeneity compared to the heterogeneity of the Canadian population.

Another approach is to look at studies that used strong methodologies with different populations to see if some association is found. Four large RCTs conducted in different settings to determine the cholesterol-lowering effect of four different drugs found an increased rate of suicide and violent deaths in each group.[1] The findings did not reach statistical significance in any of the studies, but having the findings replicated in four studies strengthens the hypothesis that there may be an association between cholesterol-lowering drugs and adverse psychologic effects. If two of the four studies had found this effect and the other two found the opposite, then there would be less reason to further consider the hypothesis. Consistent but relatively weak associations found in many studies using methodologies of varying strength will add strength to the argument that a true association exists, depending on the number of studies and their quality. Another strategy to add strength to a series of similar studies that use small numbers of patients is to merge the studies using the method of meta-analysis to determine if a cause-and-effect relationship is sustained (see Chapter 10).

Relative Risk and Relative Odds

Relative risk (RR) and relative odds (RO) are ratios calculated to determine the strength of an association. RR should be calculated only in RCTs or cohort studies and RO in case-control studies. It may be used in the problem of smoking where there is overwhelming evidence of a cause-and-effect relationship, but it can be misleading to calculate RR and RO when the cause-and-effect relationship is not firmly established.

Using the example of men who jog compared to those who do not, you could calculate the ratio of the benefit to the jogger compared to the nonjogger using the formula in Table 5-2, but only if a convincing cause-and-effect relationship is demonstrated. It needs to be empha-

Table 5–1   Decreasing Methodologic Strength of Trials

Strongest Trials
- Randomized controlled study
- Cohort study
- Case control study
- Case series
- Descriptive study

Weakest Trials

Table 5–2   Determining the Strength of an Association

	Adverse outcome	No adverse outcome
Exercised regularly	A	B
Did not exercise regularly	C	D

Relative Risk (RR) $= \dfrac{A/(A+B)}{C/(C+D)}$ (used with RCT and cohort studies)

Relative Odds (RO) $= \dfrac{AD}{BC}$ (used with case control studies)

sized that in the absence of the raw data used in a study, RR and RO may be misleading. This will be discussed further in Chapter 6 under "Numbers Needed to Treat."

The Impact of Temporality

Another means of determining the strength of an association is to assess the appropriateness of the temporal relationships. Temporality addresses the timing of exposure to the purported cause in relation to the outcome. Superficially, one would think that temporality would be quite obvious; however, an example demonstrates that human behavior is elusive.

Excessive stress during pregnancy may cause low birth weight infants. However, mothers of low birth weight babies may smoke more, are more often involved in abusive relationships, and have a higher rate of poverty and malnutrition than mothers of normal birth weight babies.

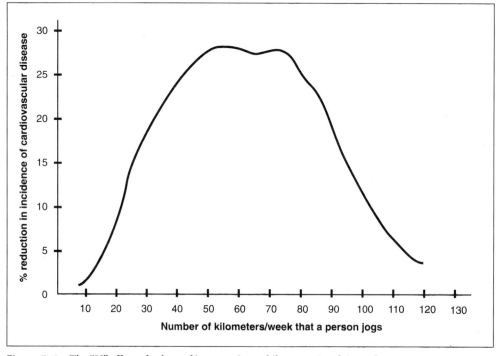

Figure 5–1   The "U" effect of a dose of intervention—kilometers/week jogged.

Each of these confounding variables could contribute to stress or may be an independent variable contributing to low birth weight. If the effects of a specific stressful event (e.g., the death of a close relative) could be assessed during different stages of pregnancy in a number of women, the time of the event may establish the temporal relationship between stress and the effect on birth weight. The timing of the introduction of the variable identified as causative in relation to the outcome becomes critical in assessing the strength of the relationship.

Dose-Response Gradient

A similar test of the strength of an association is what is known as the dose-response gradient, where an increased "dose" of the intervention is expected to yield a greater effect. If people who smoke one pack of cigarettes per day for 20 years have a 25% greater risk of dying from lung cancer, then people who smoke two or more packs per day would be expected to have a higher risk of mortality (i.e., a 30 to 40% higher risk). If jogging protects men from cardiovascular disease, do 40-year-old men who run 6 kilometers per week have incrementally more protection against heart disease than those who run only 3 kilometers per week?

A further enhancement of the dose-response curve may be the so called "U" effect. Using the jogger as an example, an overdose of the intervention (e.g., running 40 kilometers per week) may cause an increase in cardiovascular mortality. The "U"-curve arises from plotting a graph of different doses (kilometers run per week) to determine the dose at which the benefit is at a maximum and a higher dose begins to bring less benefit and becomes harmful (Figure 5–1).

Biologic Sense

If the adverse effect of a very high dose makes biologic sense (e.g., running 70 kilometers per week), then it strengthens the logic of the dose-response and further strengthens confidence in the association. However, if the "U" curve phenomenon does not make biologic sense, then support for a cause-and-effect relationship is reduced.

Epidemiologic Sense

After answering all the previous questions, one should also ask if the cause-and-effect association makes epidemiologic sense. The complexity of biologic relationships allows the possibility of an epidemiologic or biologic explanation for almost any association. Adding credibility to an association is dangerous if it is based on weak evidence from methodologically flawed studies. We are all familiar with dietary cause-and-effect relationships based on weak studies that can be quite convincingly justified by biologic, epidemiologic, or even anthropologic arguments. We know from studies assessing the effect of cholesterol lowering on mortality that those on lipid-lowering drugs have a higher rate of death overall from suicide and violence.[1] It could be argued that persons "forced" to eat a low-fat diet become angry, frustrated, and depressed. This explanation makes some sense from a biologic and anthropologic viewpoint but is not based on any scientific studies. It follows that a cause-and-effect relationship that passes assessment for validity gains strength if it also makes biologic and or epidemiologic sense. This point further emphasizes the importance of the specific sequence in which questions are asked in the assessment of a cause-and-effect relationship. Even when an assessment of a cause-and-effect relationship survives questions answered in the correct sequence, a cause-and-effect relationship is still not assured. It is very difficult to make specific cause-and-effect relationships between consumption of a specific food and specific health outcomes, yet few weeks pass without some "authority" attempting to do so.

TEACHING / LEARNING TIPS

- Select a topic raised by a patient about an association and explore the cause-and-effect relationship to determine whether the relationship can be supported.

- Take any cause-and-effect claim that is currently being promoted and review the material on which the claim is made.

- Ask students to justify a cause-and-effect relationship they believe to be true.

- Hold a seminar after students have reviewed this chapter to discuss cause-and-effect relationships and how patient questions can be answered.

- Have students keep a list of all questions raised by patients about cause-and-effect relationships.

- Have students document all assumptions about cause-and-effect relationships used in the clinical setting by both clinicians and patients.

- Use the above list as the basis of a seminar where the students do searches and critiques of the literature to determine the basis for commonly assumed cause-and-effect relationships.

Historical Support for Cause and Effect

The credibility of a cause-and-effect relationship can often be enhanced not only by methodologically sound studies but by observation, experience, and historical evidence as well. An example might be the relationship between consumption of charcoal-broiled foods and cancer. Both animal studies and cohort studies of individuals with long-term exposure to hydrocarbons have identified carbon and hydrocarbons as being carcinogenic. If a reasonably sound cohort study met all the criteria arguing for a cause-and-effect relationship, then our historical knowledge about hydrocarbons as carcinogens would add strength to the association between eating charcoal-cooked food and the development of carcinoma of the stomach. However, the historical argument supporting an association should only be used after all the other questions have been answered, and never used, as we see frequently in the media, as the principal justification. "Authorities" often use the historical argument without other criteria for an association being met. In the authors' experience, the most frequently asked questions from patients about cause-and-effect relationships deal with food consumption. It is clear that strong cause-and-effect relationships linking outcomes with consuming specific foods are extremely difficult to support in an evidence-based way. Review Chapter 16.5 for the importance of expert opinion over evidence.

QUESTIONS TO ASK WHEN REVIEWING STUDIES DEMONSTRATING A CAUSE-AND-EFFECT RELATIONSHIP

1. Does the article being reviewed deal with a POEM or a DOE?
2. How strong is the methodology?
3. Were the comparisons made on appropriate groups? Did the patients used in the comparison represent a population comparable to the practice population?

4. Were all relevant outcomes of the study measured? Were the measurements valid and described in a way that would be reproducible?
5. Was the analysis appropriate? Did the analysis include consideration of confounding variables?
6. Is the association strong? What is the relative risk?
7. Is there replication of the findings in several studies? Is the association reasonably consistent between studies?
8. Is the temporal relationship correct?
9. Is there a dose-response relationship?
10. Does the association make biologic and epidemiologic sense?
11. Is the association limited to a single cause and effect?
12. Is the association supported by historical relationships?
13. Is there enough evidence of a cause-and-effect relationship to begin to advise patients to change their behavior?

SUGGESTED ARTICLES TO EVALUATE

Ekelund LG, Haskell WL, Johnson JL, et al. Physical fitness as a predictor of cardiovascular mortality in asymptomatic North American men. N Engl J Med 1988;319(21):1379–1384.

Meanwell CA, Kelly KA, Wilson S, et al. Young age as a prognostic factor in cervical cancer: analysis of population-based data from 10,022 cases. Brit Med J 1988;296:386–391.

RECOMMENDED READING

Department of Clinical Epidemiology and Biostatistics, McMaster University. How to read clinical journals: IV. To determine etiology or causation. Can Med Assoc J 1981;124:985–989.

Richardson WS, Detsky A. Users' guide to the medical literature. How to use a clinical decision analysis: Are the results of the study valid? JAMA 1995;274:570–574.

Fletcher RH, Fletcher SW, Wagner EH. Clinical Epidemiology—The Essentials. Baltimore: Williams and Wilkins, 1996:228–248.

REFERENCES

1. Canadian Task Force on the Periodic Health Examination. Periodic health examination, 1993 update: 2. Lowering the blood/total cholesterol level to prevent coronary heart disease. Can Med Assoc J 1993;148(4):521–537.

Will a Medical Intervention Meaningfully Benefit a Patient?

As to disease. Make a habit of two things—to help or, at least, to do no harm.
Hippocrates

The intrinsic expectation of most physician-patient encounters is that the meeting will result in an action that will improve the patient's health. Of the thousands of medical therapies available today, few have been evaluated in a way that clearly identifies whether the intervention is beneficial or harmful to the patient. This chapter provides a method of evaluating the medical literature to determine if a proposed intervention is likely to do the patient more good than harm.

Key terms used in this chapter are Type I error, Type II error, contamination, transparency, statistical significance, and clinical significance. Consult the glossary for definitions.

LEARNING OBJECTIVES

Upon completion of this chapter the reader should be able to

1. determine if a proposed intervention is applicable to his/her patients;
2. determine if an intervention is likely to do more good than harm; and
3. apply strategies to help patients determine if a therapy is good or bad for them, taking into account their own life situations and values.

THE BENEFITS OF MEDICAL INTERVENTIONS

Physicians are highly motivated to alleviate the suffering of those who seek their advice when ill and in distress. In any physician-patient encounter, particularly when new symptoms are present, the patient expects the physician to provide therapy. Given this pressure, most physicians feel compelled to do something concrete by the end of the visit. It is not surprising that most physicians are more comfortable providing patients with a requisition for physiotherapy or a prescription for medication than they are telling patients they have a self-limiting disorder that will disappear even without therapy.

Patients' expectation to receive a prescription as the outcome of a physician encounter is formally acknowledged in government clinics in Hong Kong, where each individual pays for a prescription prior to the physician encounter. Given the large number of therapeutic interventions currently available and this expectation for therapy, Hippocrates' statement "primum non nocere" (at least to do no harm) carries even more meaning today than it did 2500 years ago.

Primum Non Nocere

It is essential that physicians are continually reminded that every intervention carries with it both risks and benefits. An example of what physicians perceive as a noninterventionist therapy, but which actually has potential to do more harm than good, is bed rest. Most of us have experienced the weakness that occurs after several days in bed with a bout of influenza. Undoubtedly, the fever or infection that kept us in bed contributed to the weakness, but each week spent in bed results in a loss of muscle mass of approximately 3%. Even the muscle mass lost in several days requires 1 or 2 weeks for recovery.[1] For a frail elderly person, this could represent loss of independence or a significant reduction in mobility.

Patients suffering an acute low back strain were traditionally advised to rest in bed for 5 days and then mobilize slowly. This advice was found to be counterproductive in two randomized controlled trials.[2,3] The trials found that minimal or no rest, and continuous mobilization, even if painful, resulted in a more rapid recovery and return to work than the traditional directive of bed rest. The management of low back pain has been carefully analyzed by the Agency for Health Care Policy and Research (AHCPR) to produce evidence-based guidelines that are practical for use in clinical practice. More detailed advice about low back pain based on the AHCPR guidelines can be found in Chapter 18.2.

To receive approval in a western country (especially in the U.S. and Canada), a new drug must have extensive evaluation, including a double-blind RCT before being released into the market. The agent with which the new drug is compared in these trials is important, as new drugs may demonstrate no advantage over conventional treatments, and may be more costly. These trials should be reviewed by the practitioner. Therapeutic interventions other than drugs may be introduced without evaluation. Some of these procedures become so widely accepted that appropriate evaluation through an RCT is considered unethical because it would deprive some patients of potential benefit. For example, the practice of inserting tympanostomy tubes in the ears of children with chronic otitis media was introduced without evaluation, and became widely accepted as the standard of care. Attempts to mount RCTs were considered unethical because they would deprive the control group of this accepted standard. Fortunately, an RCT is being conducted and the preliminary results question the benefit of inserting tympanostomy tubes in all but a few children with chronic otitis media.[4] A three-year follow-up study has demonstrated poorer hearing in children with tubes compared to those who went untreated.[5]

THE RCT AND BIAS

Although a randomized controlled trial is the strongest methodology to reduce bias, it can have some weaknesses (see Chapter 4). The most prevalent of these are:

Selection Bias

The most effective way to control selection bias is to randomly allocate individuals into groups to either receive the intervention or serve as a control. Extensive patient selection usually occurs before random allocation so that trial participants may differ from family and general practice.

Type I and Type II Errors

A randomized controlled trial must have a sufficient number of participants enrolled in each group for the investigation to be meaningful (Type I error). Follow-up must be adequate or a Type II error will result. For example, a two-week follow-up of 75-year-olds using a new nonsteroidal anti-inflammatory drug may not demonstrate the potentially serious side effect of gastrointestinal bleeding, which tends to occur at 4 to 6 weeks of use. Because of cost and other difficulties in conducting long-term follow-up, short-term studies with small numbers are the rule rather than the exception.

Contamination

Clinicians should identify possible contamination of the intervention or control groups in a study. After randomization, investigators must ensure that people in the control and intervention groups are not exposed to anything that could indirectly affect the genuine difference(s) between the two groups. Accidental exposure of any control group members to the intervention will artificially narrow the difference between the intervention and the control groups, thereby increasing the risk of producing a Type II error in the conclusion. An example of contamination in a study is the allocation of members of the same family to control and intervention groups in a study involving dietary modification.

When considering a new therapy, at least one carefully conducted RCT, or preferably more than one methodologically strong RCT should have demonstrated that the therapy provides clinically significant benefits to populations comparable to those in their practice. All RCTs should be transparent and should include a clear description of when randomization occurred and the criteria used to randomize the patients. New interventions not supported by evidence from replicated RCTs should be treated with caution.

Outcomes in RCTs

On occasion, a widely accepted therapy may turn out to be more harmful than beneficial (e.g., bed rest for low back pain). When evaluating the quality of an RCT, ensure that all important outcomes of therapy are reported. Investigators with a specific viewpoint may report only those outcomes which support their viewpoint.

Methodological pressures imposed by rigorous RCT methods pressure researchers to measure only DOE outcomes when a clinician's interest is in the POEM. The concepts of POEM and DOE are important in deciding whether the appropriate outcomes are being measured from the viewpoint of clinical practice.

The POEM and DOE strategy can be used to look at the ongoing discussion over screening and treatment for hypercholesterolemia. Cardiologists and lipidologists argue that the most important outcome in determining the effect of therapy is the percent decrease in serum cholesterol, or the modification of the LDL to HDL ratios. They cite evidence from the Framingham study* which demonstrates a clear link between higher levels of serum cholesterol and higher mortality rates over more than 20 years of follow-up.[5,6]

The assumption is that lowering of serum cholesterol should lower the mortality rate. This assumption has not been supported when all-cause mortality is measured in cholesterol-lowering studies. Most studies have less than 10 years of follow-up, providing the argument that 10 to 20 years are required. Another error in assumptions is found in the first large trial on cholesterol lowering, known as the NCEP trial, which involved only employed men working for a large company in the United States. The results of this study were extrapolated (and still are) to include women.[7] All subsequent major studies on cholesterol lowering that have included women have failed to show any significant benefit.[8]

Reducing dietary fat intake is widely accepted as desirable and beneficial in lowering cholesterol. The Los Angeles Veterans Study followed a group of veterans in a chronic psychiatric hospital (not likely generalizable to clinical practice) who were randomized to one of two groups: one group received an average North American diet with 40% or more fat content, and the other group received a diet of less than 30% fat content. The cholesterol and

---

* Framingham study — There are many reports and materials that have stemmed from the longitudinal follow-up of the residents of Framingham over the past 30 years.

lipid profiles of individuals in the low-fat-diet group improved within weeks of the onset of the study and remained lower for the duration of the study. However, no difference in mortality rate between the two groups was found after 8 years of follow-up.[9]

The Los Angeles Veterans Study remains the best evidence of the benefits of a low-fat diet. We should allow these little-discussed findings to temper the vigor with which we give dietary advice that may result in significant changes in lifestyle and quality of life, not only for the individuals we are advising but also their families. If the outcome measure is the DOE (lower cholesterol), then a less-than-30% fat content diet is effective. However, if the outcome is a POEM (mortality and quality-of-life issues), we are still waiting for the evidence of benefit.

The use of lipid-lowering drugs is more controversial than dietary advice. In four RCTs assessing the effect of different drugs on lipid lowering, all four drugs, cholestyramine, colestipol, gemfibrozil, and pravastatin, significantly reduced serum cholesterol (up to 29%) and demonstrated varying effects on the low-density lipoprotein (LDL) and high-density lipoprotein (HDL) profiles. The study results demonstrated a significant reduction in coronary events and a reduction in fatal heart attacks with lipid lowering. However, all four studies demonstrated that when determining all-cause mortality (the POEM) there is an increase in death from other causes, including violent death and suicide, that neutralizes the reduction of coronary deaths. In the colestipol study, the mortality rate in the intervention group was significantly higher than in the control group.[10] Although all of these trials were rigorously conducted RCTs involving large cohorts, the results are subject to wide-ranging interpretation.[11,12]

Advocates of drug interventions choose the DOE as the endpoint of a study, arguing that cholesterol reduction significantly reduces the number of cardiovascular events; they cannot understand why anyone would question this benefit. They argue that none of these trials was designed to consider all-cause mortality as an outcome, and that measuring it creates a Type I error. The evidence-based group argues that the clinically relevant outcome (the POEM) is mortality and the results of four RCTs fail to demonstrate any reduction in all-cause mortality. POEM supporters also point out the increase in violent deaths and suicides in each study implies that cholesterol and lipid-lowering drugs have psychological effects and that a conservative approach to lipid lowering seems prudent.

The good news in the cholesterol debate is that two large randomized trials that were POEMs demonstrated a benefit from cholesterol lowering using pravastatin or simvastatin in specific groups of people. In the Four S trial, men and women aged 55 to 70 years treated after a cardiac event (secondary prevention) with simvistatin to lower their cholesterol to 5.5 mmol/L showed a benefit. In the West Scotland Study, men aged 45 to 65 years whose cholesterol was greater than 7.0 mmol/L benefited from screening and primary prevention interventions with the cholesterol-lowering agent pravastatin.[14] These findings suggest all individuals who have suffered a coronary event should have their cholesterol assessed, and that men 45 to 65 years of age should also have their cholesterol levels assessed to determine if they would benefit from pravastatin therapy. We await evidence of benefit in other groups, especially women, to whom investigators may be tempted to extrapolate these recent findings.

When the representative of a pharmaceutical company, or anyone else, tries to convince physicians that a new therapy is beneficial or superior to the current therapy, it is critical that the most clinically important outcome of the intervention be delineated. If relevant clinical outcomes from the family and general practitioner's viewpoint have not been measured, then the results should be rejected. Relevant outcomes must also include consideration of quality of life. Although treatments for chronic conditions may not improve life expectancy, if they improve the patient's quality of life, they deserve consideration.

Clinical and Statistical Significance

When evaluating a study to determine whether results did more good than harm, debate often centers around the importance of statistical and clinical significance. Statistical significance is usually reported as $p = 0.05$, meaning the results of the study have less than a 5% chance of being incorrect. An important consideration about statistical significance is that the calculation is influenced by the number of people in the study. In large studies involving thousands of people, small differences between the control group and the intervention group (e.g., 3%) will be significant. To illustrate this point, in a pilot study 50 people who have pharyngitis are randomly allocated to one of two groups; one group receives a placebo drug and the other receives the active drug. Fifteen of the 25 enrolled in the treatment group recover from the condition within three days, but only 12 in the placebo group recover in the same period. These findings would not be statistically significant at a $p = 0.05$ level because of the small numbers. However, with evidence from this pilot study, funding is provided for 4000 individuals to be randomly allocated to one of two groups, resulting in 1500 patients in the intervention group and 1400 in the placebo group recovering within three days. The large cohort makes the results of this study statistically significant because it is unlikely the difference occurred by chance alone.

Both statistical and clinical significance should be considered. A 3% improvement, as in the above example, although statistically significant, is unlikely to be *clinically* significant in most situations.

Clinical significance is a judgment about whether an intervention brings enough benefit, compared to potential harm, to warrant its recommendation. The information should be presented to the patients so that they may decide for themselves. Would a potential 3% increase in the chance of shortening the course of an illness be worth a cost of $55? The answer of a senior citizen living on a pension might be quite different from that of a business executive. The socioeconomic demographics of a practice will influence the adoption of new interventions, especially those of marginal benefit.

Accounting for All Entering an RCT

When evaluating a study proposing a new intervention, it is important that all persons who entered the study at the time of randomization are accounted for at the end. Every longitudinal study has dropouts or individuals lost to follow-up and researchers should document the reasons for dropping out. The physician will have to judge if the numbers of dropouts and their reasons make the study invalid (see Chapter 4).

Table 6–1   Relative Risk and the WHO Clofibrate Study

Drug Recipients			Control
5,331			5,296
	Number of cardiac events		
131	Relative risk	.75	174
	Number of deaths		
36	Cardiac relative risk	1.05	34
40	Cancer relative risk	1.19	24
18	Violence relative risk	1.47	15
92	Other relative risk	1.74	53

RELATIVE RISK AND NUMBERS NEEDED TO TREAT (NNT) OR HARM (NNH)

Table 6–1 outlines the results of the WHO clofibrate study in which 10,627 men between the ages of 45 and 60 were randomly allocated to receive or not receive clofibrate. Of 5,331 men taking clofibrate, 131 men suffered a cardiac event, compared to 174 of 5,296 men in the control group who suffered a cardiac event.[12] A pharmaceutical representative marketing clofibrate would argue that there was a 2.55 times reduction in the relative risk of a cardiovascular event in those taking the drug. However, to put this argument in context, 43 (174–131) of the 5,331 men who took 25 mg of clofibrate daily and followed a strict low-fat diet for more than 5 years were able to avoid a cardiac event when compared to the control group. Is this a clinically significant benefit? Furthermore, the all-cause mortality numbers show that 41 more men died in the treatment group than in the control group.

Because RR and RO (see Chapter 5) can be abused by pharmaceutical companies exaggerating the benefit of an intervention, it is helpful to look at the real issue for clinicians, which is how many people do we need to treat and for how long, to get the benefit (NNT) or cause harm (NNH).[15]

The statistician calculates how many patients would need to receive the treatment or intervention for one patient to receive one unit of benefit or harm. A unit could be a life-year saved or lost, a quality life-year gained or lost, or any other measurable outcome, preferably a POEM.

The formula used to calculate the NNT or NNH from a study is:

$$1/(X-Y)$$

where X and Y are the percentage event rates with and without the intervention.

If persons with diastolic blood pressures between 115 and 129 mm Hg are treated with antihypertensives for $1^{1}/_{2}$ years, bringing their diastolic pressure below 90 mm Hg, only three people need to be treated to avoid a death, stroke, or myocardial infarction. For people whose diastolic blood pressure is between 90 and 109 mm Hg, 128 people require $5^{1}/_{2}$ years of treatment to avoid one death, stroke, or myocardial infarction.[16] (See Appendix on page 176.)

This strategy provides a useful way of deciding whether a procedure is of value to patients and useful for one's practice and helps you avoid taking RR and RO at their face value. The numbers needed to clearly demonstrate benefit or harm from an intervention may also give meaning to difficult concepts, providing simpler explanations for patients.

Assessing a new intervention using these tools will enhance confidence about the introduction of a new therapy. Generally, few studies proposing new drugs or therapies meet these stringent criteria. Most students reviewing the literature find that of the thousands of articles published, only a few survive the rigors of evaluation as described. Another strategy for dealing with the many new therapies proposed is to be conservative and allow a new therapy to be marketed for several years before considering its use. This approach may deprive patients of beneficial new therapies. By asking the outlined questions, physicians can avoid the pitfalls of adopting a new therapy that does more harm than good, while quickly adopting the therapies that will be beneficial.

The Patient's Perception of Benefit Versus Risk

Once the benefits and risks of a therapy are understood, each patient's views must be taken into account. The PPPP asks the patient to consider a therapy in the context of their own values. When the patient's views are included in the final partnership agreement, the use of evidence for optimum individual benefit occurs (see Part II).

TEACHING / LEARNING TIPS

- Select a frequently prescribed medical intervention and review the evidence of benefit on which the treatment was based.

- Select a therapy that a patient has questioned as a result of recent media coverage, and critique the article on which the therapy is based.

- On the next visit of a pharmaceutical representative, ask for the literature supporting claims for the drugs and assess them using the outlined questions.

- At the next continuing education event, when a therapy is recommended, ask for the literature that supports the therapy and critique it.

- Ask students to define and discuss the concepts of contamination of a study, Type I error, Type II error, and statistical and clinical significance.

- Ask students to use the low back pain PPPP when treating a patient with an acute low back strain, and evaluate those guidelines which reduce the risk of doing more harm than good.

QUESTIONS TO ASK WHEN REVIEWING ARTICLES ON THE BENEFIT OF THERAPY

1. Is the proposed therapy a POEM or a DOE?
2. Was the randomization to treatment and control groups explained in a transparent and reasonable fashion?
3. Were the patients in the study comparable to your practice population?
4. Were all important outcomes described?
5. Were both clinical and statistical significance appropriately dealt with in the study?
6. Is the proposed therapy feasible in your practice setting?
7. Were all patients who entered the study accounted for at the end of the study?
8. How will this study impact on your practice?

SUGGESTED ARTICLES TO EVALUATE

Williams JW, Holleman DR, Samsa GP, Simel DL. Randomized controlled trial of 3 vs. 10 days of trimethoprim/sulfamethoxazole for acute maxillary sinusitis. JAMA 1995;273:1015–1021.

Shepherd J, Cobbe SM, Ford I, Isles CG, et al. Prevention of coronary heart disease with pravastatin in men with hypercholesterolemia. N Engl J Med 1995;333(20):1301–1307.

RECOMMENDED READING

Fletcher RM, Fletcher SW, Wagner EH. Clinical Epidemiology: The Essentials. Third Edition. Baltimore, MD: Williams & Wilkins, 1996. pp.136–164, 165–185.

Levin MS, Walter SS, Lee HN, et al. Users' guide to the medical literature. 4. How to use an article about harm. JAMA 1994;271:1615–1619.

REFERENCES

1. Ferrando AA, Stewart CA, Bruwder DG, Hillman GR. Changes in muscle volume during seven days of strict bedrest. Aviation, Space and Environment Medicine 1995;66(10):976–981.

2.   Lahad A, Maiter AB, Berg AO. The effectiveness of four interventions for the prevention of low back pain. JAMA 1994;272:1286–1291.

3.   Nachemson AL. Newest knowledge of low back pain. A critical look. Clin Orthop 1992:p. 279.

4.   Maw R, Bawden R. Spontaneous resolution of severe chronic glue ear in children and the effects of adenoidectomy, tonsillectomy, and insertion of ventilation tubes. Brit Med J 1993;306(6880):750–760.

5.   Viannel WB, Castelli WP, Gordon T. Cholesterol in the prediction of atherosclerotic disease. New perspectives based on the Framingham study. AWN Intern Med 1979;90:1985–1991.

6.   Viannel WB. High density lipoproteins: Epidemiologic profile and risk of coronary artery disease. Am J Cardiol 1983;52:9B–12B.

7.   The Lipid Research Clinics Coronary Primary Prevention Trial results: 1. Reduction in incidence of coronary heart disease. JAMA 1984;251:351–364.

8.   The Task Force on the Periodic Health Examination. The Canadian Guide To Clinical Preventive Health Care. Ottawa: Minister of Supply and Services, 1994;650–671.

9.   Dayton S, Pernice M, Hashimoto S, et al. A controlled clinical trial of a diet high in unsaturated fat in preventing complications of atherosclerosis. Circulation 1969;40(Suppl 1):1–63.

10.   Dorr AE, Gunderson K, Schneider JC, et al. Colestipol hydrochloride in hypercholesterolemic patients. Effect on serum cholesterol and mortality. J Chronic Dis 1978;31:5–14.

11.   Frick MH, Elo O, Haapa K, et al. Helsinki Heart Study: primary prevention trial with gemfibrozil in middle aged men with dyslipidemia. Safety in treatment, changes in risk factors, and incidence of coronary heart disease. N Engl J Med 1987;317:1237–1245.

12.   Report from the Committee of Principle Investigators. A co-operative trial in the primary prevention of ischemic heart disease using clofibrate. Br Heart J 1978;40:1069–1118.

13.   Scandinavian Simvastatin Survival Study. Randomized trial of cholesterol cornering in 4444 patients with coronary heart disease. Lancet 1994;344(8934):1353–1389.

14.   Shepherd J, Cobb SM, Ford I, et al. Prevention of coronary heart disease with pravastatin in men with hypercholesterolemia. West of Scotland Coronary Prevention Group. N Engl J Med 1995;333(20): 1301–1307.

15.   Cook RJ, Sackett D. The numbers needed to treat—a clinically useful measure of treatment. BMJ 1995;310:452–454.

16.   MRC Working Party. MRC trial of treatment of mild hypertension: principle results. Br Med J 1985;291(6488):97–104.

CHAPTER 7

How to Determine if a Therapy is Cost Effective

One of the first duties of the physician is to educate the masses not to take medicine.
Sir William Osler

During the last half of the twentieth century, health care costs became a major component of the economy of every developed country. With health care expenditures accounting for 14% of the United States' gross national product (GNP), 9% of Canada's, and 8% of most European countries', the economic implications are significant. There is evidence that increasing expenditure on health care does not equate with improvement in the health status of the population. The World Bank has demonstrated that improving employment and housing, and narrowing a country's economic gap between the rich and the poor will make a greater contribution to improved health than building more hospitals or increasing expenditures on health care.[1]

Key terms used in this chapter are viewpoint, input, output, efficacy, cost analysis, cost-effectiveness, cost-minimization, cost-effectiveness analysis, cost utility, and discounting. Consult the glossary for definitions.

LEARNING OBJECTIVES

Upon completion of this chapter the reader should be able to

1. better understand the terminology of economic analysis;
2. use the methods described to determine the cost-effectiveness of a medical intervention; and
3. review a paper on cost-effectiveness and determine if the conclusions apply to clinical practice.

Economic factors play an important part in deciding on one treatment over another. However, the terminology and methodology used by economists are often unfamiliar to physicians. This chapter explains the terms and approach used in economic analysis to evaluate a therapy, allowing you to make an evidence-based judgment when considering an intervention. All economic analysis studies should be preceded by studies which show that the intervention is effective, efficient, and feasible.

TERMINOLOGY OF ECONOMIC ANALYSIS

Viewpoint

Every economic analysis should be considered from multiple points of view, e.g., government, insurance company, hospital, physician, and patient. If a district health council is asked to spend $200,000 on a new piece of physiotherapy equipment on the basis of evidence that demonstrates major savings in time lost from work, it would argue from the viewpoint of the overall economy, employers, physicians, and the individual. The viewpoint of the hospital budget officer would be significantly different; his or her agenda is to operate the hospital more efficiently in a time of diminishing resources. The physiotherapy equipment would increase operating costs and provide minimal benefit for only a few hospital employees. A new laundry machine which would save $400,000 annually would have greater priority. In the discussion of any economic analysis, all viewpoints should be included along with a description of the impact of each perspective (Table 7–1).

Input and Output

Input refers to an estimate of all identifiable costs incurred in implementing a program. Output refers to the most complete estimate possible of the human and financial benefits that will accrue from an intervention, e.g., all POEM and DOE outcomes in addition to the economic outcomes. Economic analysis should compare the input and output of alternative interventions.

Cost Analysis and Cost-Minimization Analysis

A cost analysis is a study that examines only the cost of potential alternatives. A cost analysis of the use of two different rubella vaccines to immunize women and subsequently prevent rubella syndrome in the newborn would assess only the cost of the vaccines and their administration. Cost minimization analysis would compare the cost of immunizing in physicians' offices to immunizing in public health clinics.

Cost-Effectiveness and Cost-Benefit Analysis

In cost-effectiveness analysis a unit value is assigned to all the POEM and DOE outcomes and the costs are examined. The analysis may also be done by comparing all input costs against a common outcome, such as comparing the input costs of two rubella immunization programs (physicians' offices vs. public health) using the dollar cost per case of rubella syndrome prevented as the common outcome.[2]

Cost-benefit analysis is used when comparing two different programs with different outcomes, for instance, the effect of lipid lowering on the rate of heart attacks compared to the

---

Table 7–1   Types of Costs and Consequences Used in Economic Evaluation

Costs

Direct
1.   Organizational costs (health care, professional time, capital costs, supplies and operating costs)
2.   Costs borne by patients and their families, including all out-of-pocket expenses

Indirect
1.   Time lost from work
2.   Emotional stress

Costs to Society
1.   All costs outside of the health care system and the family.

Consequences

1.   Changes in physical, emotional, or social function.
2.   Changes in resource use (health benefits).
     Improvement in operating and organizing health care services for the original condition and unrelated conditions. Changes relating to families such as savings in lost time costs or savings in work time lost.
3.   Changes in the quality of life for patients and families (utility)

effect of immunization programs on disability. This is difficult because it involves attaching a dollar value to both the interventions and the outcomes. Analysis includes not only the dollar cost per unit of outcome but also the dollar value of the number of days of disability suffered, medical complications avoided, marital disruption reduced, prevented episodes of depression, and other difficult-to-measure parameters. A monetary value must be assigned to life, life events, and emotional and physical function. One of several problems associated with cost-benefit analysis is the lack of validated measurement scales for quality of life, marital discord, the impact of various medical complications, or the impact of an adverse drug reaction on the quality of life.

Cost-Utility Analysis

Cost-utility analysis addresses the perceived value of an improvement in health status for an individual, a specific group, or society in general, in other than monetary terms. Utility is measured by determining the preferences of individuals and society for specific health outcomes and is affected by the individual's perspective. For example, a fracture of the fifth digit is inconvenient to a truck driver, but devastating to a concert pianist.

The interesting contribution of the concept of utility is that the measurement uses a unit known as quality adjusted life year (QALY) which allows for comparison of different interventions with different outcomes (Table 7–2). This provides valuable information to assist in resource allocation.

Discounting

Most preventive interventions done now will lead to a beneficial effect only after many years have elapsed. A future benefit is not a sure thing because of factors such as accidents or disease, and therefore is not worth as much as an immediate benefit. Hence, economists discount the value of interventions at a rate of 2 to 10% per year as they calculate cost benefit.

A study has demonstrated that a 55-year-old male taking 80 to 100 mg of ASA daily will lower his risk of myocardial infarction by 30% over 10 years.[3] To develop a cost analysis for taking daily ASA, the estimated cost of a one-year supply of ASA is $100. The cost of a myocardial infarct is estimated at $2,000 per quality of life year lost. Over 10 years, taking ASA would cost $1,000. The purchasing power of $1000 in 10 years will not be equal to $1000 today. The economist would point out that the value of an immediate benefit from an intervention occurring today is greater than spending the money now and not receiving any benefit for 10 years. The declining value of the upfront expenditure during the 10 years of

Table 7–2   Treatment Costs per QALY*

Treatment	Cost/QALY (Aug 1990)
Cholesterol testing and diet therapy (all adults aged 40–69)	£ 220
Advice to stop smoking from general practitioner	£ 270
Antihypertensive treatment to prevent stroke (ages 45–64)	£ 940
Breast cancer screening	£ 5,780
Cholesterol testing and treatment (incrementally) all adults aged 25–39	£ 14,150

*Adapted from Mason J, Drummond M, Torrance G. Some guidelines on the use of cost-effectiveness league tables. BMJ 1993;306:570–572.

waiting for benefit needs to be discounted when doing the economic analysis. If all the ASA were purchased now, the $1,000 investment would be discounted at the average rate of about 5% per year (the discounting rate is different than the inflation rate). Discounting rates are usually established in the literature or by government as between 2 and 10%. Over 10 years the value of the investment would decline, as would the value of the benefit. The dollar difference between cost and benefit would decrease, making the cost-benefit of the strategy less attractive.

Incremental Analysis

When analyzing the benefit of a new program, determining its incremental cost of implementation is useful. An example of this is the evaluation of a lipid screening program. The cost of measuring serum cholesterol in men aged 45 to 59 years who have one or more cardiovascular risk factors (obesity, hypertension, or smoking) can be compared to screening all men in this age group. From this information, a cost-utility analysis could be developed which compares men with and without risk factors. If a full lipid profile was then done on both groups, the incremental cost and incremental benefit of this procedure could be determined. Assessing the incremental cost of adding more complex but reasonable procedures and comparing the benefit added with each increment should be part of a complete economic analysis.

Sensitivity Analysis

Sensitivity analysis refers to the assessment of the economic impact of the various assumptions on which an analysis is based, such as per diem costs, discount rates, etc. The more complex the analysis, the more assumptions are made. A sensitivity analysis examines costs and benefits in the best and worst case scenarios. It tests the impact of changing the discount rate to 2%, 3%, 4%, 6%, or 7%. If a 1% change in the discount rate changes a program from being cost effective to becoming cost ineffective, then the benefits are marginal.

LIMITATIONS OF ECONOMIC ANALYSIS

Economic analysis assumes the effectiveness, efficiency and availability of a program. It often limits itself to cost or benefit within the health care budget and not in other areas like the work force, education, or housing. It implies that money saved in one area will be redistributed to other areas, which may or may not occur. Assumptions rarely account for factors such as the anxiety that occurs while awaiting test results. Family and general physicians are aware that the shift of health care from the hospital to the community will increase the need for care to be provided by family members, mainly women. How do economic analyses account for this effect? More economists are talking about the need to take into account "human capital." These complexities create difficulties in accounting for all assumptions made in economic analysis.

One also needs to ask whether the analysis applies to an individual practice or community. Are the values underpinning the analysis clear and well described, and do they reflect the values of the community? Has the analysis broadened the understanding of how decisions could be made, and clarified the possible choices?

APPLICATION OF ECONOMIC DEFINITIONS

The greatest value in achieving an understanding of the basic terminology used in economics will be in the ability to critically assess proposals from hospitals or community bureaucracies. Some basic questions will need to be asked about the quality of economic analysis to determine the relevance of such proposals and whether they deserve further consideration.

TEACHING / LEARNING TIPS

- Choose two different approaches to common office tests such as thyroid screening or cholesterol testing, and ask students to develop a list of all possible costs involved.

- Using the first example, generate a comprehensive list of all the benefits from the test or procedure.

- Ask students to determine how they would calculate costs and benefits in a way that would allow comparisons.

- Make students aware of the costs of different drugs and investigations that they order in clinical practice.

- Ask students to look at the side-effect profile and benefit profile of several different drugs and determine what measures of quality of life are needed for comparison.

- Review the terminology used in economic analysis (definitions).

- Review a paper with students that analyses a drug or procedure that you use, asking the questions about the quality of the analysis.

- Encourage discussion about the cost of tests, procedures, or referrals made in clinical practice.

- Review a profile of your own test ordering, prescribing, or referral patterns, if available, considering the cost-effectiveness. What measures are needed to accurately assess cost-effectiveness using practice profiles?

The questions asked in any economic analysis must be clear, answerable, and classified as dealing with a POEM or a DOE. The effectiveness of a well-defined intervention should have been established by a randomized controlled trial or a cohort study. If the answer to any of these questions is negative, then further assessment of the analysis is unnecessary.

The question must include current costs and costs of alternatives. All costs must be included, not only those that accrue in an institution but the actual costs to the payer (insurance company or Ministry of Health), the cost to the institution and the health care providers involved (including physicians), and the cost to the patient and family in expenses, lost income, and the loss of personal time. An example of the application of economic analysis in deciding the value of a proposed intervention can be found in the Chapter 14.4, where home monitoring of uterine activity to prevent preterm births is evaluated.

Given the complexities involved in measuring all relevant costs of medical interventions, it is unrealistic for a family and general practitioner, unless specifically trained, to be able to make these judgments. It is essential that the family and general practitioner be satisfied that all costs from their viewpoint (practice and patients') have been documented. (A more detailed discussion of health economic instruments can be found in reference 1.) A health economist may be consulted about the quality of the instruments used in an analysis under consideration. Assuming that appropriate measurement instruments were used, the experienced clinician can make a judgment about the credibility and value of the results. Attaching a dollar value to quality of life or life years saved allows the comparisons needed to decide on the most appropriate therapeutic intervention. Clinical judgment about the accuracy of the assumptions made in the analysis also provides a valuable perspective, allowing assessment of their applicability to clinical practice.

QUESTIONS TO ASK WHEN REVIEWING AN ECONOMIC ANALYSIS

1. Is the proposal dealing with a POEM or a DOE?
2. Is the question clear and answerable?
3. Is there strong evidence of benefit from the intervention?
4. Were all costs and effects of the intervention considered, including all important viewpoints and all reasonable alternatives, including doing nothing?
5. Were appropriate and comparable units used to measure costs or benefits in the analysis?
6. Were costs and benefits discounted and adjusted in a reasonable way?
7. Was an incremental analysis of all costs and benefits performed?
8. Was a sensitivity analysis performed?
9. Did the analysis make sense from your viewpoint? Give reasons for your answer.
10. How will this study impact on your practice?

SUGGESTED ARTICLES TO EVALUATE

Frame PS, Fryback DG, Paterson C. Screening for abdominal aortic aneurysm in men ages 60 to 80 years. J Fam Pract 1993;119(5):411–419.

Van der Mass PJ, deKoning HJ, Van Ineveld BM, et al. The cost-effectiveness of breast cancer screening. Int J Cancer 1989;43:1055–1060.

RECOMMENDED READING

Department of Clinical Epidemiology and Biostatistics, McMaster University. How to read clinical journals: VII. To understand an economic evaluation (Part A). Can Med Assoc J 1984;130:1428–1434.

Department of Clinical Epidemiology and Biostatistics, McMaster University. How to read clinical journals: VIII. To understand an economic evaluation (Part B). Can Med Assoc J 1984;130:1542–1549.

Sackett DL, Richardson WS, Rosenburg W, Haynes RB. Evidence-Based Medicine. New York: Churchill Livingston, 1997;142–145.

REFERENCES

1. Evans RG. Strained Mercy: The Economics of Canadian Health Care. Toronto: Butterworth and Co. Canada, 1989.

2. Steering Committee of the Physician's Health Study Research Group: Preliminary report: Findings of the aspirin component of the ongoing Physician's Health Study. N Engl J Med 1988;318:262–264.

CHAPTER 8

Will This Review Article Help Me to Better Understand My Patients' Problems?

Nature fits all her children with something to do.
He who would write and can't write, can surely review.
James R. Lowell

For several decades review articles have been seen as the salvation of the family and general practitioner. Most journals designed for family and general practitioners use review articles as one of their main features. The purpose of this chapter is to assist in the assessment of the quality of a review article to determine if its conclusions should influence your behavior.

LEARNING OBJECTIVES

Upon completion of this chapter the reader should be able to

1. determine if the question asked by the review article is appropriate;
2. determine if the process of producing the review was adequately rigorous to consider using the conclusions; and
3. decide if the review is applicable to the patients.

ASSESSING THE QUALITY OF REVIEW ARTICLES

Most review articles combine the clinical experience of the author and their personal review of the literature. As the concept of systematic critical review of the literature evolves, expert opinion is no longer considered to be firm enough evidence on which to base practice changes. As with all other evidence-based approaches, there are standards for review articles that are designed to reduce the potential for bias.

The Question

In a properly done review article, the methods must be so transparent that any physician could replicate the process and arrive at similar conclusions. The question to be answered by the review should be clearly stated at the start. If, at first glance, the question is unclear or confusing, there is little point in reading further. A clear question should address three elements: 1) What population is being dealt with in the review? (the clinician's question is, how well does the population relate to my practice?) 2) What is the intervention being dealt with in the review? (the clinician's question is, is the intervention something you would or could do in your practice?) 3) What is the outcome sought for in the review? (the clinician's question is, is the outcome a POEM or a DOE?).

If these three elements of the question are not clearly addressed upfront, or even if they are clear but the answers to the clinician's questions suggest that there is a problem with relevence, then it is unlikely that the article's conclusions will apply to your clinical practice.

Many review articles do not address specific questions but provide a broad overview of a problem or condition. The traditional review describes the etiology, signs, and symptoms of a problem such as low back pain, and goes on to describe the author's approach to diagnosis and management using a few selected references. From an evidence-based perspective, this style of review article has some value in providing an expert's approach to a common problem, but the methodology is not rigorous enough to ensure that the conclusions represent an objective and systematic review of the current literature.

The Literature Search

The sources of data used in the search, including key words, personal communications with researchers, discussions at scientific meetings, or other less formal sources of information, should be described. The transparent literature search techniques should use key words that are relevant to the question(s).

There have been studies conducted which suggest that the literature tends to be biased in favor of the publication of positive results. Another documented bias is towards prominent authors whose publications are accepted in preference to those of unknown authors, despite similar rigor in design, methodology, and outcome of studies.[1] Thus, the published literature may not always reflect all the current knowledge about a specific question. Investigators in a research project supported by a pharmaceutical company who discover higher rates of side effects than have been reported previously may never submit their findings for publication, creating another form of publication bias.

It is not possible for the author of a review article to overcome all these obstacles, but highlighting them does illustrate the importance of a rigorous search strategy, and the deficiencies of even the most rigorous search. The search description should show that a reasonable effort was made to obtain all relevant literature in an attempt to reduce bias as much as possible. The author should then discuss the criteria for inclusion or exclusion of literature and demonstrate that the process of decision making was as objective as possible. The inclusion and exclusion criteria must be stated so clearly that if other independent reviewers applied the same search criteria they would choose the same primary papers. The author of a rigorous review should report that an independent reviewer using the same criteria and search strategy did indeed choose the same articles.

Amongst the criteria for selecting an article should be the study's population, the interventions, and the outcomes that were considered for inclusion or exclusion. It is important to determine if the outlined criteria make sense in family and general practice.

The decision to include or exclude articles on the basis of study methods used is also important. The stronger the study methods demanded in the review, the greater confidence there can be in the conclusions. Most rigorous reviews include only randomized controlled trials in their search; however, this strategy risks not addressing important questions for family and general practice.

When rigorous criteria are used, even if hundreds or thousands of studies have been published on a subject, usually only five or ten papers will meet the criteria. Although it is rare to find a review article that is rigorous about the literature selection, all reviews that do not follow the prescribed level of rigor are at risk of bias. An example of biased paper selection can be drawn from the cholesterol debate, where inclusion or exclusion of papers greatly influences the conclusion of a review. If the endpoint considered in a review is cholesterol lowering, then a number of well-controlled randomized trials demonstrated success for a number of widely prescribed drugs (a DOE rather than a POEM).

Assessment of Quality of the Literature

Once the primary studies to be included in the review have been selected, the author must then review the quality of the studies. An assessment of this process will use all the skills acquired from understanding Chapters 1 to 7. The review should include a brief commentary on the strengths and weaknesses of each primary study. The commentary on each selected article should include the numbers and characteristics of the population, the duration of the study, the outcomes and how they were measured.

These brief descriptions give the reader a sense of the strength, quality, and relevance of the studies from which the review has drawn its conclusions. There should be evidence that the critique of the primary studies was objective. Objective and unbiased reviews are best achieved by having two or three individuals review and critique each article independently and then share their opinions. If the results of the studies chosen by the author for inclusion are inconsistent, then the possible causes of the inconsistency should be discussed. There are five components of a clinical study where minor differences can result in different outcomes:

1. the study design,
2. chance,
3. the population used,
4. the intervention used, its duration and strength, and,
5. the way in which outcomes were measured.

If the review uses randomized controlled trials, cohort studies and case-control studies, the potential for bias in the methodologically weaker studies is likely to provide some explanation for variability of outcome. If the sample sizes in the studies are small, chance may play a major role in the variability of results. The student's t-test and measurement of confidence limits are the common way to assess the risk of chance alone accounting for the results. The smaller the sample size the less likelihood of a difference being statistically significant and the more likely a difference can be explained by chance alone. Chance may explain minor differences between studies, but large differences in outcome are more likely to be explained by the population sample. Often, factors such as the severity of illness of patients in two samples will explain a difference. Difference in the age or sex distribution of the study samples or racial differences in the two populations are factors that might explain differences. Study outcomes may differ because of dosage differences, or different rates of compliance. Outcome measures may vary from one study to another, especially in those measuring quality of life as an outcome, where both the instruments and the methods by which the information is gathered may vary. An example of a critique of the literature that uses review articles as the basis of the conclusions of the critique can be found in Chapter 14.5 on assessing the use of electronic fetal monitoring during labor.

Combining Data in a Review

It may be reasonable in a rigorous review to merge the results from several of the key studies using the techniques of meta-analysis (Chapter 10). The author may use meta-analysis techniques to bring the results of several small studies together. If only some studies are merged, you should query why a full meta-analysis was not carried out using all available comparable studies.

If meta-analysis is not appropriate, then the author should produce a table with the most important characteristics of each of the primary studies displayed in a way that makes comparisons between each study clear. Assuming all studies are randomized controlled trials, then the table might include the numbers of persons involved in each trial, the interventions, comments on the methodology and differences in outcomes. If all the findings are consistent, then this may be helpful in supporting a conclusion. If the results are conflicting, with some

TEACHING / LEARNING TIPS

- Ask students to find a review article relevant to a clinical question that they have and review the article.

- Have the students review five to seven family medicine journals, collect all the review articles and then do a superficial assessment of the quality of the review articles relative to the criteria stated in the chapter.

- Get students to assess a review article from a pharmaceutical industry-sponsored publication, and identify weaknesses or sources of bias.

- Do a literature search on a clinically relevant subject. Take review articles identified in the search and determine how many meet these criteria.

- At a journal club, subject review articles used to the criteria outlined.

studies showing a positive effect and others showing a negative effect, it may be necessary to combine the results in a meta-analysis before any conclusions can be drawn.

Conclusions in a Review Article

Conclusions from a review should be based on findings from the review. This seems like an obvious statement, but there are some examples of rigorously conducted reviews that draw conclusions that are not linked to the findings of the review.[2]

Review articles are an important source of information for all primary care providers. Historically, most review articles have been opinion papers. As we approach the 21st century, opinion is no longer a sound enough basis on which to practice medicine. Primary care providers must demand rigorously constructed review articles in order to trust them as sources of information for evidence-based practice. This demand must be repeatedly expressed to the editors of journals designed to assist family and general practitioners so that the quality of review articles will continue to improve.

QUESTIONS TO ASK WHEN EVALUATING A REVIEW ARTICLE

1. Is the review about a POEM or a DOE?
2. Is the question clearly stated?
3. Was the strategy used to search the literature rigorous, unbiased, and described in a transparent way?
4. Were the criteria for inclusion or exclusion of articles explicit?
5. Was the quality of the primary articles used in the review discussed? Was a table of the primary articles' findings included? Were differences in results from the studies explained by assessing differences in methods?
6. Was meta-analysis considered? Was the rationale for using or not using meta-analysis provided?
7. Are the conclusions of the review supported by the analysis of the literature?
8. How will this review impact on your practice?

SUGGESTED ARTICLES TO EVALUATE

Assendelft WJJ, Hay EM, Ashead R, Bouter LM. Corticosteroid injections for lateral epicondylitis: a systemic overview. Br J Gen Pract 1996;46(405):209–216.

Koch B. Glucose monitoring as a guide to diabetes management. Critical subject review. Can Fam Physician 1996;42:1142–1152. (An example of current standards of review.)

RECOMMENDED READING

Oxman AD, Guyatt GH. Guidelines for reading literature reviews. Can Med Assoc J 1988;138:697–703.

Oxman A, Cook D, Guyatt G. Users' guide to the medical literature. JAMA 1994;272:1367–1371.

Oxman A, Guyatt G. The science of reviewing research. NY Acad Sci 1993;703:125–134.

REFERENCES

1.   Hutchison BG, Oxman AD, Lloyd S. Comprehensiveness and bias in reporting clinical trials. Study of reviews of pneumococcal vaccine effectiveness. Can Fam Physician 1995;41:1356–1360.

2.   Hunt RH, Mohamid AH. The current role of Helicobacter eradication in clinical practice. Scand J Gastroenterol 1994;Suppl 208:47–52.

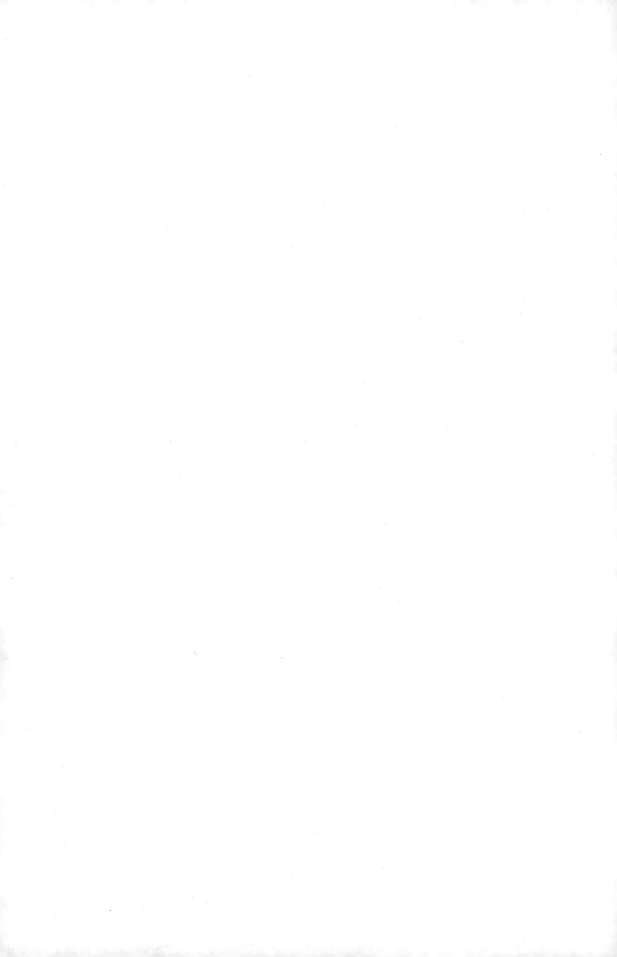

CHAPTER 9

Choosing Guidelines with Confidence

Knowledge should be his guide, not personal experience.
Plato

The 1990s could be called the decade of clinical guidelines. Many medical journals, specialty groups, and government agencies have published "authoritative" guidelines that include strong suggestions for their implementation in family and general practice. Medical specialty societies, pharmaceutical manufacturers, and food producers finance the development and publication of guidelines which attempt to influence the prescriber and consumer to adopt behavior that is beneficial to the interest group. This chapter provides a strategy to determine if a guideline is evidence-based.

Learning Objectives

Upon completion of this chapter the reader should be able to

1. distinguish a relevant guideline from an irrelevant guideline;
2. determine if a guideline has been produced using evidence-based criteria; and
3. determine if one should adopt the guideline in his/her practice.

Evidence-Based Guidelines

The idea of guidelines based on a rigorous review of the current literature is attractive. If guidelines consolidate the knowledge about complex health problems into clear action steps, then they have value. The practitioner wishing to practice evidence-based medicine needs an efficient means of assessing the quality of a guideline. The American Academy of Family Practice has developed three questions that should be asked:

1. Who produced the guideline?
2. Is the guideline relevant to family and general practice?
3. What was the approach to obtaining evidence to support the guideline?[1]

The production of high-quality guidelines is expensive and has to be paid for by someone with an interest in the topic. Any guideline that does not explicitly state who supported the cost of production and their reason for sponsoring the guideline should be considered with a healthy dose of skepticism.

Any guideline producer claiming to have an evidence-based approach should identify the members of its advisory panel, and how they were selected. Controversy has arisen over individuals who appeared unbiased but were identified as being dependent on research grants from companies with a stake in the guideline content, e.g., the N.C.E.P. guidelines.[2] A tendency to exclude family and general practitioners when structuring guideline panels, even though most guidelines are targeted at primary care providers, has also been observed. High-quality guidelines should list the members of the panel, their discipline, expertise, or qualifications, how they were chosen, and any conflict of interest they have with stakeholders in the guideline production.

When a panel member has a conflict of interest, a description of how the conflicts were dealt with should be included. Failure to provide all the above information, or mention that it is available, should make one suspect potential bias. This level of transparency and integrity is rarely found and will become more common only if guideline consumers demand it.

Questioning Guideline Production

If you ask who produced the guideline and why, the answer should identify likely sources of bias. Specialty groups may produce guidelines broadly defining their area of expertise, hoping to reduce encroachment on their "turf."[3] Pharmaceutical companies produce guidelines promoting use of their products, especially new families of drugs, by raising physician and public awareness of a health problem. Third-party payers or governments may support guideline production in an attempt to reduce cost or promote more cost-effective approaches to health care delivery. Support for guideline production by a specific interest group does not mean the guideline is necessarily biased and should be rejected.

The recommendation arising from a guideline must take into account all impacts of the recommended interventions including quality of life and economic costs. The quality of the economic analysis should stand up to the rigorous assessment outlined in Chapter 7. The clinician must assess the costs and savings likely to accrue if the guidelines are fully implemented, and be satisfied that the benefits derived from improved outcome justify the costs. A direct and robust linkage between the conclusions from the literature review and the guideline should exist. Guidelines exist which follow a rigorous and transparent path in their production but which abandon obvious conclusions to promote a predetermined recommendation.[4] In Chapter 17.3, the guidelines for screening to prevent prostate cancer are found. These guidelines generate frustration because no effective strategies are recommended. However, the review demonstrates the hazards of implementing guidelines which risk doing more harm than good.

Guidelines produced by the U.S. Agency for Health Policy Reform are rigorously produced and usually include a field trial with practitioners and subsequent modification before the final version is published.[4] Table 9–1 outlines the guideline production steps by the Agency for Health Care Policy and Reform of the U.S National Institute of Health used to produce guidelines for management of depression. Some physicians complain that this process is too cumbersome to be practical, but the steps can be justified. If sweeping recommendations with the potential to affect millions of individuals are to result from a process, then it is not unreasonable to demand a high degree of rigor.

Relevance of the Guideline

Many guidelines are produced with little or no input from family and general practitioners. They are often irrelevant to the clinical setting because they are DOEs and not POEMs, or are difficult to implement. The barriers to acceptance and flexibility to adjust the guideline according to age, lifestyle, individual preferences, etc., should be discussed.

Evidence Used in the Guideline

The principles of rigorous critical appraisal of the literature apply to guideline production. The approach to conducting the literature search and selecting the primary articles on which a guideline is based should be explicit and rigorous. The search strategy, key words used, extra materials gathered, criteria for inclusion and exclusion, and a critique of the individual primary studies used to support the guidelines must be included. A biased literature review can concentrate on the benefits of an intervention while ignoring harmful effects. Important

Table 9–1   Guideline Development Process

Topic chosen by AHCPR

Panel chair chosen by AHCPR

Panel members recommended by the chair and AHCPR

Panel convened and focus for literature reviews defined

Twenty-one diagnostic and 18 treatment topics selected for review

Literature reviewers for specific topics selected by panel

NLM literature searches conducted using key words selected for each topic by panel/reviewers with MEDLINE and Psychiatric Abstracts for each topic

Abstracts reviewed for inclusion/exclusion criteria by literature reviewers

Full copy of each article selected read by literature reviewers

Literature review and evidence tables created by literature reviewers

Review read/critiqued by panel chair, methodologist, and a minimum of three panel members

Reviews revised where indicated relevant parts of each review abstracted by panel for Depression Guideline Report

Depression Guideline Report drafted by panel

All reviews independently reviewed by all panel members and 14 scientific reviewers

Depression Guideline Report revised

Depression Guideline Report synopsized to Clinical Practice Guideline, A Patient's Guide, and Quick Reference Guide for Clinicians

Peer review requested from 73 organizations and 14 new scientific reviewers, pilot review of A Patient's Guide, Quick Reference Guide for Clinicians, and Clinical Practice Guideline in nine sites

Critiques from peer/pilot review considered by panel

All versions of guidelines reviewed by panel

Final copy of all versions of guidelines submitted to AHCPR

undesirable side effects of an intervention such as anxiety or behavioral change may not be discussed. If evidence is conflicting or confusing, a meta-analysis of good quality should be carried out as part of the guideline production (see Chapter 11).

QUESTIONS TO ASK WHEN REVIEWING GUIDELINES

1. Is the guideline dealing with a POEM or a DOE?
2. Who produced the guideline? What is their reason for producing the guideline?
3. Who is on the guideline panel and how were they selected?
4. Was any conflict of interest of panel members addressed and appropriately managed?
5. Was the method of literature search transparent, rigorous and comprehensive, including all relevant data?
6. Were all impacts of the intervention considered, including quality of life and cost-effectiveness?

TEACHING / LEARNING TIPS

- Identify a number of guidelines, then assess them in terms of POEMs or DOEs.

- Ask students to take several guidelines they have received, and evaluate them.

- Review an office procedure adopted because of recent guidelines, and assess their quality against the criteria in this chapter.

7. Has the feasibility of implementation in a practice similar to yours been tested or considered?

8. Would you consider implementing the guideline in your practice?

SUGGESTED ARTICLES TO EVALUATE

Canadian Thoracic Society Working Group. Guidelines for the assessment and management of chronic obstructive pulmonary disease. Can Med Assoc J 1992;147(4):420–427.

Podell RN. National guidelines for the management of adult asthma. Am Fam Physician 1992; 46(4): 1189–1195.

RECOMMENDED READING

Hayward R, Wilson M, Tunis S, et al. Users' guide to the medical literature. 8. How to use clinical practice guidelines: Are the recommendations valid? JAMA 1995;274:570–574.

REFERENCES

1. American Academy of Family Practice. Brochure on Assessing Guidelines. Kansas City: AAFP, 1994.

2. Expert Panel on Detection, Evaluation and Treatment of High Blood Pressure in Adults. Summary of the second report of the National Cholesterol Education Program (NCEP). JAMA 1993;269: 3015–3023.

3. Moore TJ. The cholesterol myth. Atlantic Monthly 1989;264(3):37–70.

4. Hunt RH, Mohamid AH. The current role of Helicobacter eradication in clinical practice. Scand J Gastroenterol 1994;Suppl 208:47–52.

5. Agency for Health Care Policy Reform. Guidelines for managing depression in Primary care.

CHAPTER 10

Evaluating the Quality of a Meta-Analysis

*Meta-analysis is the biostatistician's playpen
from which projectiles are thrown at terrorized clinicians.*
Anonymous

Meta-analysis is the process of systematically merging data from similar studies in order to clarify conflicting findings or to add strength to the findings of several small studies. This chapter will assist you in developing a strategy to determine if a meta-analysis meets evidence-based criteria and comes to conclusions that will assist in clinical decision making.

LEARNING OBJECTIVES
Upon completion of this chapter the reader should be able to

1.   determine the relevance of a meta-analysis to his/her patients;
2.   assess the quality of the meta-analysis to determine if the conclusions are valid; and
3.   be confident the results of the meta-analysis are appropriate for his/her practice.

WHY DO A META-ANALYSIS?
Merging the results of several RCTs may provide information that cannot be obtained from each study independently. Small trials, although less difficult and less expensive to carry out, are subject to Type II error (i.e., false negative results occurring by chance). Pooling of the results from several similar RCTs reduces the risk of Type II error and strengthens confidence in the conclusions. A further benefit can be derived from pooling results from analyses of subsets from larger trials. In the past few years subsets of persons representing specific age/sex groups or a group with unique characteristics have been derived from very large trials in order to answer specific questions applicable to these smaller groups. The numbers in these subset analyses are small. Pooling the results strengthens the statistical power of the analysis.

The risk of a Type I error (i.e., false positive results occurring by chance) also exists in small trials. Pooling data from all the trials reduces this risk. Another possible advantage to pooling several small trials, compared to results from one large trial, is that the sampling bias of the large trial is minimized by the differences in the samples from several small studies. The meta-analysis of a number of small trials should be more generalizable to family and general practice populations than results from a single large trial.

One area in which meta-analysis has aided the family physician in decision making is in hormone replacement therapy for women (Chapter 18.7).

ASSESSING THE QUALITY OF META-ANALYSIS

The Question
The question being asked by the meta-analysis must be clear. One should decide if the question is a POEM or a DOE. If the question sustains your interest, then attention must be paid to whether the trials can be combined. Trials to be included in a meta-analysis are usually chosen from a carefully conducted literature search for RCTs which ask the same question.

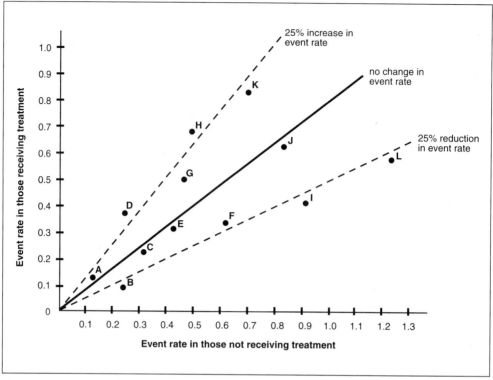

Figure 10–1 An example of heterogeneity of a number of studies (not suitable for meta-analysis).

The rules for a transparent literature search (Chapter 8) should be followed. The authors should state why they decided that meta-analysis was necessary. Reasons might include the impracticality of conducting a large enough single trial to answer the question, the presence of small trials or subset analysis and the absence of a large trial, and the importance of the question in health care delivery. Often a series of small trials have results that are inconsistent and by combining them a more definitive conclusion is possible.

Once the literature, both published and unpublished (publication in progress or preliminary data pending publication), has been assembled with an explicit description of the inclusion and exclusion criteria used, the authors should provide a description of the characteristics of each trial included in the meta-analysis. An example of unpublished literature that carries significant value can be found in Chapter 15.4 on otitis media, which contains information from a trial not yet published. The detailed description of each trial is usually displayed in a table and includes the type of intervention, dose, duration of treatment, and the characteristics of the patients in the trial relevant to the intervention. A description of the methods used including the point of randomization and a description of the outcomes for both the trial and the control groups should be included.

Assessing the Methodology of Studies

Once the reviewers have assembled and described the studies to be included in the analysis, they need to provide a quality score for each study. At least two independent reviewers score each study based only on its methods. The reviewers should be blind to the authors and other identifying characteristics of each study. This is easier said than done as panel members are usually familiar with the literature. Differences in the quality scores between reviewers should be discussed.

Merging the Results of Trials

Trials can only be merged when the outcome measures used in each trial are consistent. Variations in the results of the studies should correspond to differences in the characteristics of the studies. An "eyeball" estimate made by the reader should correspond to an estimate of the magnitude of difference between the intervention and the control when the trials are combined.

Homogeneity

If the combined studies are comparable, variation in their outcomes should be accounted for by sampling variation or chance. The results can be demonstrated graphically by plotting the control groups along the horizontal axis and the intervention groups along the vertical axis. Significant variation suggests a lack of homogeneity in the studies being merged indicating that combining their results is inappropriate (Figure 10–1). Although a number of statistical tools are available to analyze homogeneity (Mantel and Haenszel equation),[1] one's own judgment about homogeneity from the plot is a simple way to determine if combining the studies is appropriate. Lack of homogeneity may reflect different doses of the intervention or different age/sex composition of the study populations. Table 10–1 demonstrates a homogeneous set of trials that can be appropriately combined. A good meta-analysis gives you a table like this and explains any differences.

Sensitivity Analysis

Sensitivity analysis responds to the question: Are the results of the meta-analysis sensitive to changes in the way in which the analysis is done? An example would be to conduct a meta-analysis using only RCTs and then to add cohort studies that otherwise meet the same criteria,

Table 10–1 Trials on the Effect of Lipid Lowering Strategies (the effect of cholesterol lowering on cause-specific and all-cause death rates)

Trial	Cardiac	Non Cardiac	Cancer	Violence	Total
Drug Trials					
LRC	0.78	1.34	1.06	2.75	0.96
HHS	0.84	1.30	0.99	2.48	0.96
WHO	1.05	1.74	1.66	1.19	1.47
UCS	0.59	1.60	1.00	5.00	0.62
Total	0.88	1.54	1.32	1.77	1.14
Diet Trials					
LAUDS	0.80	1.06	1.70	9.04	0.96
MCS	1.39	1.00	1.34	1.50	1.00
Total	0.90	1.02	1.55	1.79	1.00

Adapted from the Canadian Task Force on Periodic Health Examination. 1993 update. Lowering the total blood cholesterol to prevent coronary heart disease. Can Med Assoc J 1993;148:521–537.

TEACHING / LEARNING TIPS

- Ask students to review a meta-analysis that addresses a question arising from clinical work.

- Ask students to list questions raised from seeing patients or from patients' questions. Ask students to search the literature for review articles or meta-analyses that address these questions. Have a meeting to discuss the quality of the literature.

- Review a meta-analysis recently reported in the media against the criteria to see if the findings are applicable to your practice.

- Scan journals to find a meta-analysis. Scan that analysis for the characteristics discussed in this chapter. If the analysis passes the rapid scan, then answer the detailed questions about the paper.

- Critique an analysis that has changed your practice behavior in the past few years.

to see if the outcome changes. A similar outcome after combining studies using different methodologies adds confidence to the meta-analysis results. Age or sex groups might be excluded from combined data as a strategy to measure their influence in determining outcomes. The results of this type of sensitivity analysis may strengthen confidence in the meta-analysis if the results make clinical sense, and confirm clinical observations.

After reviewing a meta-analysis and determining that the analysis has been carefully conducted and meets the outlined criteria, one can be confident the results are relevant and useful for patients. Although statisticians may lose our attention in areas within the process of meta-analysis (the actual mathematical process of pooling the data), the general principles of good meta-analysis can be judged by any clinician. Many meta-analyses in the literature do not meet the above criteria, so the mathematical wizardry becomes irrelevant.

QUESTIONS TO ASK WHEN ASSESSING THE VALUE OF A META-ANALYSIS

1. Is the question a POEM or a DOE?
2. Is the question clearly stated?
3. Is the literature search strategy described in a transparent fashion?
4. Are there explicit inclusion and exclusion criteria and an appropriate explanation for the studies that were included?
5. Is homogeneity of the studies appropriately evaluated?
6. Are appropriate statistics used? Is sensitivity analysis used?
7. Does the pooled analysis demonstrate significant differences between the trial and control groups?
8. Are appropriate conclusions drawn from the analysis?
9. Would you incorporate the recommendations into your practice?

SUGGESTED ARTICLES TO EVALUATE

Romero R, Oyarzun E, Mazor M, et al. Meta-analysis of the relationship between asymptomatic bacteriuria and preterm delivery/low birth weight. Obstet Gynecol 1989;3:576–582.

Steinburg KK, Thacker SB, Smith SJ, et al. A meta-analysis of the effect of estrogen replacement therapy on the risk of breast cancer. JAMA 1991;65(15):1985–1990.

RECOMMENDED READING

Egger M, Smith GD. Misleading meta-analysis [editorial]. BMJ 1995;310:752–754.

Felson DT. Bias in meta-analytic research. J Clin Epidemiol 1992;45(8):885–892.

Jeng GT, Scott JR, Burmeister LF. A comparison of meta-analysis results using literature vs. individual patient data. Paternal cell immunization for recurrent miscarriage. JAMA 1995;274:830–836.

Naylor CD. Two cheers for meta-analysis: Problems and opportunities in aggregating results of clinical trials. Can Med Assoc J 1988;138:892–895.

Sacks HS, Berrier J, Reitman D, et al. Meta-analysis of randomized controlled trials. New Engl J Med 1987;316(8):450–455.

REFERENCE

1.   Dawson-Saunders B, Trapp RG. Basic and Clinical Biostatistics. East Norwich, CT: Appleton-Lange, 1994:189.

CHAPTER 11

Assessing a Study on Quality of Care

Come, give us a taste of your quality.
Hamlet
William Shakespeare

Professions are self-regulating bodies granted special privileges by society with the expectation that they share their knowledge and expertise to benefit society. Practitioners are responsible to their regulating bodies and their patients for the quality of their work. This chapter reviews evaluation strategies for quality of care studies with particular attention to assessing quality in primary care practices.

LEARNING OBJECTIVES

Upon completion of this chapter the reader should be able to

1. use the methods described to assess studies on the quality of medical care;
2. determine the relevance of these studies to his/her practice; and
3. decide if the introduction of a quality of care measure would be beneficial to patients.

ASSESSING PRACTICE QUALITY

The care being assessed should have been shown by at least one RCT to result in a POEM benefit. Three aspects of care are usually assessed in quality assurance studies:

1. the *structure* of the overall health care system and of the caregiver organizations;
2. the *process* of providing the care; and
3. the *outcomes* of the care.

All three aspects—structure, process, and outcome—must be addressed in a quality-of-care article. Studies including only one or two of these components are of questionable value.

The System Structure

The structure of the overall health care system refers to organization and financing of a system at a national or local level and includes a description of the guiding principles of that health care system. The percentage of gross national product invested by a country in health care may be included. Outcome measures are usually at the macro level using indicators like longevity, maternal mortality and perinatal mortality rates.

Quality measurements at a practice organization level usually document the qualifications of the providers, the physical and technical facilities available, and the organizational structure in which the providers work. Most quality assurance studies occur in settings that differ considerably from an individual physician's practice environment. Each practitioner will have to decide what these differences mean to their interpretation of the study's results.

Process of Providing Care

All the steps relevant in history taking, physical examination, diagnostic testing, and therapy should be included. This does not imply an endless checklist of process steps but a comprehensive and practical list of criteria representing all aspects of care. Unfortunately, the results of quality assurance studies do not support the idea that a clinician who is excellent at history taking will also be an excellent diagnostician or an excellent administrator of therapeutic interventions. This is why all aspects of care and potential barriers must be considered.

Studies have demonstrated that 15 to 20% of process steps carried out by the physician are not recorded in the medical record, and yet many quality-of-care assessments depend on them as the source of measurement. The method of measuring the process of care should be unbiased, objective, and transparent. Evaluators should be blind to the physician and patient participants and even to the specific process steps being measured.

Measuring Outcomes

Inappropriate measuring of outcome carries risks. If the outcome is infrequent in general and family practice, one might conclude that positive or negative events do not occur (Type I error). For instance, it is likely that fewer than 10 diagnoses of malignant melanoma will occur in a 30-year practice career. Measuring the outcome of a melanoma screening program over 5 years in an individual practice could be misleading, with the possibility that no such events are recorded. If a prevention program has a delayed outcome (e.g., early detection of abnormal cells by Pap smear to prevent cancer of the cervix 15 to 25 years later), then assessing the outcome during a 10-year period will lead to incorrect conclusions about the effect of the screening program (Type II error).

If the outcome measure is mortality, the infrequency of that event in most practices makes its value as a quality measure meaningless unless large numbers of practices are involved in the study. Of more relevance in family practice is measurement of quality of life, function, and patient satisfaction. During the past decade, validated measurements of function have been developed for primary care practice which provide a practical way to measure important and relevant patient outcomes.[2]

When measuring outcomes, especially those involving function or quality of life, the assessor should be blind to whether patients belong to the study group. If functional status is being measured as the outcome of a quality assurance assessment of a rehabilitation program, then administration of the functional status measurement instrument should be conducted by an individual from outside the study environment. All outcomes must be measured including social support, cost-effectiveness, quality of life, and patient satisfaction. All deaths or drop-outs from treatment must be identified so that every entrant can be accounted for. For patients lost to follow-up, the worst outcome should be assumed.

Improvement in outcome must achieve both statistical and clinical significance to influence a change in process of care. The basic question is: Does the improvement in quality of care resulting from the intervention justify the cost and effort required for implementation? Few quality-of-care studies meet stringent criteria, and it will be a rare event when a physician is persuaded to alter the process of practice because of the findings in one of these studies. As experience with quality-of-care studies in family and general practice increases, we may find ourselves under increasing pressure to alter procedures or tests in a "cost-effective" way. The ability to demand the evidence for such changes and assess the evidence supporting benefits of the interventions should protect clinicians and their patients from adoption of inappropriate cost-saving procedures.

TEACHING / LEARNING TIPS

- Ask a student to review an audit performed in the office or hospital using the criteria outlined.

- Find a quality-of-care report in a journal, and have a student review it against the criteria.

- Determine if two or three audits provided by the hospital meet the criteria.

- With students, plan an audit to be conducted using the criteria in this chapter.

- Pick a topic, do a literature search, find a quality assurance article, and measure its quality against the criteria.

- Choose a quality-of-care issue to address in the office and design steps using the outlined criteria. Decide whether the study is practical. Would a computerized record system help?

A good example of an important measure of quality of care in family and general practice is the effectiveness of blood pressure control in patients over 65 (Chapter 16.2). The guidelines for blood pressure control have changed significantly in the past 5 years. Monitoring the percentage of elderly people in one's practice who have an annual blood pressure check and then comparing the percentage of those whose blood pressure is higher than the recommended level is a good measure of the quality of care one provides to seniors.

QUESTIONS TO ASK WHEN ASSESSING ARTICLES ABOUT QUALITY OF CARE

1. Was the topic and outcome measure a POEM or a DOE?
2. Is there at least one RCT demonstrating benefit?
3. What was the method of selection of the health professionals described in the study?
4. Were the health professionals selected representative of your practice? Were the qualifications and the practice settings adequately described?
5. Was the workload of the practice described comparable to your practice?
6. Did the study focus on what you actually do in your practice?
7. What method was used to select patients for the study? Do the patients reasonably correspond to those in your practice?
8. Was the diagnosis described in such a way that you could easily identify inclusion and exclusion criteria for your own patients?
9. Were patients described in terms of comorbidity?
10. Were criteria for the process of care practical and transparent?
11. Did the study consider all relevant outcomes?
12. Were statistical and clinical significance considered in measuring outcomes?
13. How will this study have an impact on your practice?

SUGGESTED ARTICLE TO EVALUATE

Borgeil AEM, Williams JI, Anderson GM, et al. Assessing the quality of care in family physicians' practices. Can Fam Physician 1985;31(4):853–862.

RECOMMENDED READING

Department of Clinical Epidemiology and Biostatistics, McMaster University. How to read clinical journals: VI To learn about the quality of clinical care. Can Med Assoc J 1984;130:377–384.

REFERENCES

1.   Rosser WW, McDowell I, Newell C. Use of reminders for preventive procedures in family medicine. Can Med Assoc J 1991;145(7):807–813.

2.   McDowell I, Newell C. Measuring Health. Second edition. New York: Oxford University Press, 1996.

CHAPTER 12

Teaching and Learning about Evidence-Based Medicine

Education is not preparation for life; education is life itself.
John Dewey

Having reviewed the methods for selecting relevant literature about family and general practice and learning how to determine if the information is supported by good quality evidence, how can we effectively convey this knowledge to colleagues, residents, and medical students?

LEARNING OBJECTIVES

Upon completion of this chapter the reader should be able to

1. understand strategies for teaching and learning about the practice of evidence-based medicine in the clinical setting; and
2. formulate a plan for sustained teaching and learning about evidence-based family and general practice.

ATMOSPHERE

Probably the most powerful way to teach the principles of evidence-based medicine is to create a suitable environment in which to do clinical work. Most medical student and family and general practice resident teaching takes place in clinical settings where an evidence-based approach to practice can be modeled.

Those of us who have attempted to meet this challenge have been accused of making evidence-based practice "life itself" by questioning everything suggested in the clinical setting. One important aspect of this style of practice is to admit that one does not know the answers to many or most of the questions asked. Creating a safe atmosphere in which one is encouraged to question and reflect makes learning fun. One should be careful to not overwhelm learners but to stimulate them to be curious about the basis for interventions being suggested.

Relevant questions can be generated in the clinical setting by the clinician or student keeping a list of questions that arise in each office session. Such a list could be used subsequently for more detailed reviews. Another source of questions is the chart review carried out with students or residents at the end of a clinical session. Insightful questions are often asked by patients and learners. When the answer is unknown, it is all right to admit this and to commit to find the answer in the literature and discuss it at a later date. This search can be done by the learner alone, or together with faculty and/or the patient.

THE JOURNAL CLUB

Once relevant and important questions have been identified by a patient, clinical teacher, or learner, they can be addressed in a variety of ways to maximize the learning impact. Many clinicians and learners find journal club meetings an effective way to address questions emerging from clinical practice. Journal clubs have several advantages over conducting literature searches and critiques individually. By having a structure and fixed time of meeting there is some assurance that the reviews will actually be done. Having a group of people involved reduces the workload for each individual. Discussing the outcome of a literature review with colleagues has an advantage, given the paucity of existing clear answers, especially for questions emerging from family and general practice.

The group can collectively consider the best way to interpret the literature in the practice context and determine how to adapt the findings of a relevant study to their clinical environment. Recent evaluation of small group continuing medical education (CME) demonstrates that a problem-based small group learning session is one of the most effective ways to change physician practice behavior.[1] Although this strategy has been used since the 1880s (when first described by Sir William Osler), using evidence-based strategies in the journal club instead of opinions and anecdotes is a more recent approach.[2]

THE COURSE

Many teaching programs for family and general practice residents conduct courses in critical appraisal or evidence-based medicine. One risk of this approach is that the material is presented in a formal and didactic way, detaching the content from its clinical relevance. Asking learners to read the theoretical material before the discussion and then concentrating on the actual critique of the literature, especially if the articles are chosen by the learners based on questions arising from their clinical experience, should be an effective strategy to prevent the course from seeming unconnected to clinical practice. Another approach is to have the learners select and prepare the critique in advance and present it to their colleagues for discussion. The tutor can facilitate the process by assisting in the choice of paper for critique.

It may be helpful to use material emerging from the Cochrane Collaboration[3] and books such as The Canadian Guide to Clinical Prevention[4] which are very transparent in the way they apply critique principles.

ROUNDS

Educators may demand that when cases are presented at rounds or other regular functions the literature reviews used should always be adequately critiqued. This strategy is doomed to failure if one is the lone voice seeking this level of rigor. Ideally, all staff will be knowledgeable about evidence-based approaches to medicine, supportive of a high standard of critical review, and be willing to meet the standard when making their own presentations.

HAVING AN IMPACT ON YOUR COLLEAGUES

One individual can change the thinking of a group of physicians by using an evidence-based approach in his/her presentations. Picking a controversial issue and demonstrating how a review of evidence assists with clinical decision making may help to stimulate interest. Promoting the questioning of anecdotal or poor-quality literature may lead to colleagues asking for more information about an evidence-based approach. The questions, topics, and papers to be reviewed should arise out of issues important to the participants. The topics covered in this book could be the focus for some sessions.

REFERENCES

1.   Davis DA, Thomson MA, Oxman AD, Haynes RB. Changing physician performance: A systematic review of the effect of continuing medical education strategies. JAMA 1995;274:700–705.

2.   Osler W. Aquinamitas. Third edition. London: Macmillan, 1905.

3.   Oxman A, Chalmers I, Clark EM, et al. Cochrane Collaboration Handbook. Oxford: Cochrane Collaboration, 1994.

4.   The Canadian Task Force on the Periodic Health Examination. The Canadian Guide to Clinical Preventive Health Care. Ottawa: Minister of Supply and Services, 1994.

CHAPTER 13

Teaching and Learning with Patients: The Physician-Patient Partnership Papers (PPPP)

Most of the studies reviewed demonstrated a correlation between effective physician-patient communication and improved patient health outcomes.
Moira Stewart

How can we use the information derived from the process of critically appraising the literature for the optimum benefit of our patients? There are probably few challenges in family practice greater than trying to convince a patient that a requested diagnostic test or medication is not beneficial and may even be harmful.

LEARNING OBJECTIVES

Upon completion of this chapter the reader should be able to

1. understand the physician-patient partnership; and
2. be prepared to utilize the physician-patient partnership papers in clinical practice.

THE PHYSICIAN-PATIENT PARTNERSHIP

The concept of finding common ground is based on a growing body of literature that emphasizes the importance of the physician-patient relationship. Evidence from studies of patient-centered medicine suggests the best patient compliance occurs in an environment of collaboration and information sharing.[1] The Institute of Medicine in its definition of primary care identified a "sustained partnership" as being an essential ingredient of primary care practice.[2] Patients are dissatisfied when questions are not answered and when they do not feel that they are partners in the therapeutic decisions.[3] Leopold also documented the fact that physicians have difficulty carrying through the concept of a sustained partnership in the confines of daily practice. Table 13–1 outlines the features of a sustained partnership, and Table 13–2 lists the measurable outcomes of a sustained partnership, some of which have already been found to contribute to improved health outcomes.[3] Table 13–3 outlines the areas of a good physician-patient relationship which have been shown to lead to a benefit in health outcomes.

One demonstrated benefit involves the negotiation, acceptance, and understanding of the implications of an intervention. Achievement of the finding of common ground between physician and patient results in significantly better patient compliance with regimen requirements.[4,5] Think of the physician and patient encounter as a meeting of two coinvestigators or partners on a research project. The physician brings to the project expertise on the medical issues, while the patient is the expert on his/her experience with the disease and its effect on his/her life and values. The negotiation should involve melding evidence-based medical knowledge with the patient's experience and values as much as possible. The outcome should be satisfactory and committed to by both parties.[5] Based on the growing body of knowledge

Table 13–1 Features of a Sustained Partnership between Physician and Patient in Family and General Practice

Whole Person Focus
The family and general practitioner attends all health-related problems either directly or through collaboration regardless of the nature, origin, or organ system involved.

Physician Knowledge of the Patient
The family and general practitioner knows the person, their family, their community, their context. The physician also has knowledge and respect for individual values and personal preference.

Caring and Empathy
The family and general practitioner demonstrates interest, concern, compassion, sympathy, empathy, attentiveness, sensitivity, and consideration.

Patient Trust of the Physician
The patient believes that the physician's words are credible and reliable. The physician will always act in the patient's best interests and provide support and assurance.

Appropriately Adapted Care
The family and general practitioner tailors treatment to the patient's goals and expectations as well as patient beliefs, values, and life circumstances.

Patient Participation and Shared Decision Making
The family and general practitioner encourages patient participation in all aspects of care, treatment, and referral. To the degree the patient wishes or desires, they are involved in all decision making.

Adapted from Leopold, et al., 1996

about the importance of patient-centered medicine and its benefits, we believe that effective implementation of evidence-based medicine will require as much acceptance by the patient as it does by the physician.

THE PHYSICIAN-PATIENT PARTNERSHIP PAPER (PPPP)

In an attempt to complement these concepts, the authors have developed the PPPP. The first step in using this form is to clarify the question being asked to the satisfaction of both parties. Then the remaining sections can be completed together at that visit or the appropriate sections can be completed separately by each partner and blended at the next visit.

Table 13–2 Measurable Outcomes of a Sustained Partnership between Physician and Patient

Patient Outcomes
1. Short Term: Satisfaction, knowledge, reduced level of anxiety, intent to adhere to advice.
2. Intermediate Term: Behavioral change, adherence to program, self-efficacy.
3. Long Term: Improved physiological, functional, and behavioral health status, symptom resolution, disease prevention, reduced anxiety level, and improved quality of life.

Physician Outcomes
Improved satisfaction, accuracy of diagnosis, reduced malpractice claims, appropriateness of treatment, and patient loyalty.

Health System Outcomes
Reduced visitation, costs, reduced malpractice claims, roster stability, provider turnover.

Adapted from Leopold et al., 1996

Table 13–3   Elements of an Effective Physician-Patient Discussion about the Management of a Health Problem

Physician's Role in Facilitating Discussion
Patient encouraged to ask questions
Patient is successful in obtaining desired information
Patient is provided with information packages and programs
Physician provides clear information and emotional support
Physician willingness to share decision making with the patient
Both physician and patient agree about the nature of the problem and the need for follow-up
Measured Effects on Patient Outcomes
Reduced anxiety, reduced role limitation, reduced physical limitation
Improved functional and physiological status
Improvement in pain control, function, mood, and reduced anxiety
Reduced psychological distress, improved symptom resolution
Reduced patient anxiety
Acceleration of problem and symptom resolution

Adapted from Stewart, 1995

The physician partner's task is to use current guidelines or recommendations to outline the literature evidence of benefit or harm from the procedure or medication, and assist the patient in compiling pertinent information about their past and present health and family health.

The patient partner and their companion, where applicable and desired by the patient, are encouraged to read the summary of the evidence and consider and record their own feelings and beliefs about the evidence. This, ideally, should be done in their own context, taking the appropriate amount of time to do so on their own.

At a follow-up visit, discussion takes place. Given the background work, the discussion should be reasonably brief. A decision is negotiated and recorded. A follow-up plan is put in place. This is particularly indicated in situations where new evidence may be forthcoming. The patient takes one copy of the PPPP and one copy remains on the chart.

Part II of this book provides the PPPP for 26 issues commonly encountered in family and general practice. The discussion of the literature upon which the evidence is based can be photocopied and given to the patient for their perusal. Patients wishing even more information can be given the source articles or texts to review.

RECOMMENDED READING

Stiggelbout AM, Kiebert GM. A role for the sick role: patient preferences regarding information and participation in clinical decision making. Can Med Assoc J 1997;157(4):383–389.

REFERENCES

1.   Bass MJ, Buck C, Turner L, et al. The physician's actions and the outcome of illness in family practice. J Fam Pract 1986;23:43–47.

2. Institute of Medicine. Primary Care: America's Health in a New Era. Washington: National Academy of Science, 1996.

3. Leopold N, Cooper J, Clancy C. Sustained partnership in primary care. J Fam Pract 1996;42(2): 129–137.

4. Stewart MA. Effective physician-patient communication and health outcomes: A review. Can Med Assoc J 1995;152:1423–1433.

5. Frank E, Kupfer DJ, Siegel LR. Alliance not compliance: A philosophy of outpatient care. J Clin Psychiatry 1995;56(Suppl 1):11–15.

PART II

Applying Critical Thinking in
Family and General Practice

CHAPTER 14

Physician-Patient Partnership Papers for Pregnancy and Childbirth

14.1 PRENATAL ULTRASOUND

During the past 15 years an ultrasound examination at 16 weeks of pregnancy has become part of routine care in the developed countries. Many women with normal pregnancies will undergo two or three ultrasound examinations to help determine the expected date of birth, monitor the baby's growth, determine if there are twins, find out if the baby has abnormalities, and determine its sex. The practice of providing a copy of the ultrasound to the parents contributes to the popularity of the procedure.

What is Ultrasound?

Ultrasound uses the transmission of high-frequency sound waves to allow us to visualize the baby. The baby's head size, chest size, and leg length can be measured and estimates of the baby's stage of development can be made. At present there is little evidence of any harm resulting from ultrasound waves being transmitted through the fetus, although people continue to question the possibility of effects on hearing and other senses.

Evidence of Benefit from One Ultrasound Examination at 16 Weeks of Pregnancy

Four large studies, involving thousands of pregnant women, were conducted to compare the health of babies born to women who had a single ultrasound examination at 16 weeks of pregnancy with those who were not exposed to ultrasound.[1-4] None of the studies detected a significant difference. Four other trials measured the effect of undergoing two or more ultrasound examinations during pregnancy; the first ultrasound was done at 16 weeks, the second at 24 to 26 weeks. In some trials a third examination was done between 32 and 36 weeks of pregnancy.[5-8] None of these studies found significant differences. The largest of these studies involved approximately 7500 women undergoing ultrasound at 16 weeks and 7500 women in the control group who had undergone ultrasound only when medically indicated. Sixty-five percent of the control group did not have an ultrasound examination. This study compared the two groups for neonatal deaths, infant problems at birth including seizures, hemorrhages, need for intensive care nursing, evidence of nerve injury, a special need for oxygen, and a number of other detailed outcomes. No significant differences were found.[8]

RECOMMENDATION

The evidence does not support the use of an ultrasound at 16 weeks in a normal pregnancy.

RECOMMENDATION OF OTHERS

Many national and international organizations suggest ultrasound only when there is a specific reason and do not recommend routine ultrasound in normal pregnancy. The Canadian Task Force on the Periodic Health Examination recommends that a single ultrasound be done in all pregnant women at 16 weeks. It does not support the use of serial ultrasound.

REFERENCES

1.   Bennet MJ, Little G, Dewhurst J, et al. Predictive value of ultrasound in early pregnancy: Randomized controlled trial. Br J Obstet Gynecol 1982;89:338–341.

2.   Waldenstrom U, Axelsson O, Nilsson S, et al. Effects of routine one-stage ultrasound screening in pregnancy: Randomized controlled trial. Lancet 1988;ii:585–588.

3.   Thacker SB. Quality of controlled clinical trials. The case of imaging ultrasound in obstetrics: a review. Br J Obstet Gynecol 1985;92:437–444.

4.   Saari-Kemppainen A, Karjalainen O, Ylostalo P, et al. Ultrasound screening and perinatal mortality: Controlled trial systematic one stage screening in pregnancy. The Helsinki Ultrasound Trial. Lancet 1990;336:387–391.

5.   Eik-Nes SH, Okland O, Aure JC, et al. Ultrasound screening in pregnancy: a randomized controlled trial. Lancet 1984;i:1347.

6.   Bakketeig LS, Eik-Nes SH, Jacobsen G, et al. Randomized controlled trial of ultrasonographic screening in pregnancy. Lancet 1984;ii:207–211.

7.   Neilson JP, Munjanja SP, Whitfield CR. Screening for small for dates foetuses: a controlled trial. Br Med J Clin Res Ed 1984;289:1179–1182.

8.   Ewigman BG, Crane JP, Frigoletto FD, et al. Effect of prenatal ultrasound screening on perinatal outcome. RADIUS study group. New Engl J Med 1993;329:821–827.

Physician-Patient Partnership Paper

Patient _____

Chart I.D. _____

Physician _____

The Question: Should I have a single ultrasound at 16 weeks of pregnancy?

Information about current health, past health, and family health relevant to the question:

Medical Evidence:

Recommendation: A single prenatal ultrasound at 16 weeks does not provide benefit in a normal pregnancy.

Advantages
- early detection of significant abnormalities
- establishing accurate dates
- detects more than one baby
- reduces premature delivery
- parents get and enjoy first "baby picture"

Disadvantages
- early detection of insignificant abnormalities
- cost
- lack of evidence of outcome benefit
- detects abnormalities incorrectly leading to unnecessary intervention and anxiety
- detects normal variations causing anxiety and further tests and costs

Effect of recommendation on feelings, beliefs, values of self and family:

Physician-patient partnership decision   Date _____

Follow-up plan:

14.2   SUGAR TESTS IN PREGNANCY

Because 3% of women will have an elevated blood sugar level during pregnancy, it has become common for healthy pregnant women to be tested at 28 weeks of pregnancy. Women who are overweight, over the age of 30, or have a family history of diabetes are more likely to have elevated blood sugars. If the blood sugar is elevated at 28 weeks of pregnancy, steps can be taken to control it, thereby reducing the chance of having a large baby. Large babies tend to create obstetrical problems leading to higher birth injury and cesaren section rates. Diabetic mothers' babies may have problems with blood sugar control after birth.

The Test

Blood sugar levels are usually tested at 28 weeks of pregnancy in women with a normal pregnancy. This test involves drinking a sugar solution containing 50 or 75 gm of glucose, with blood drawn either 1 hour after drinking the solution, or before drinking the solution and then 1 and 2 hours following. If the first test is abnormal, then a second test using 100 gm of sugar in solution is carried out. Women with an abnormal second test are considered to have gestational diabetes and are treated with diet and/or insulin.

Advantages and Disadvantages

Studies have shown that treating mothers with gestational diabetes lowers the birth weight of these babies. Babies who weigh less at birth have fewer minor birth injuries, such as broken collar bones and stretched nerves in the neck. However, babies recover rapidly from both of these injuries with no long-term consequences.[1–3]

One disadvantage to testing all pregnant women is that detecting and treating elevated blood sugars in pregnancy may increase the number of babies born with a low birth weight. This, in turn, increases difficulties associated with low birth weight, such as increased infant mortality. In addition, such testing causes anxiety in the mothers, and is time-consuming and costly. Some women find the drink nauseating and the repeated blood tests unpleasant. Being identified as diabetic carries the risk of being permanently labeled as diabetic, even though only 30% of women with gestational diabetes become diabetic later in life. Thinking that one is, or may become, diabetic and having this known by insurers or employers may have undesirable implications.

RECOMMENDATION

Screening for gestational diabetes at 28 weeks is not recommended. No significant benefit to mothers or babies has been demonstrated by testing all pregnant women. The risk of low birth weight babies, erroneous labeling of women as diabetic, cost, and the unpleasant aspects of the test itself, make it difficult to justify it. The test is not recommended unless there is a high-risk situation. If the test is to be carried out, women should be informed of its limitations.

RECOMMENDATION OF OTHERS

The Canadian Task Force on the Periodic Health Examination gives gestational diabetes screening a "C" recommendation, i.e., there is poor evidence to either support or discourage the procedure. The U.S. Preventive Services Task Force recommends screening all women at 28 weeks of pregnancy with a 50 gm glucose solution.

The American and Canadian Diabetic Associations recommend testing of all pregnant women at 28 weeks.

REFERENCES

1.   Santini DL, Ales KL. The impact of universal screening for gestational glucose intolerance on outcome of pregnancy. Surg Gynecol Obstet 1990;170:427–436.

2.   O'Sullivan JB, Gelliss S, Dandrow RV, et al. The potential diabetic and her treatment in pregnancy. Obstet Gynecol 1966;27:683–689.

3.   Coustan DR, Lewis SB. Insulin therapy for gestational diabetes. Obstet Gynecol 1978;51:306–310.

Physician-Patient Partnership Paper

Patient_____

Chart I.D. _____

Physician _____

The Question:
Should I have a glucose test at 28 weeks of pregnancy to detect early diabetes?

Information about current health, past health, and family health relevant to the question:

Medical Evidence:
Recommendation: Screening for diabetes at 28 weeks of pregnancy is not recommended.

Advantages	*Disadvantages*
• will detect early diabetes	• leads to incorrectly labeling women diabetic
• leads to reduction of minor birth injuries	• leads to increase in low birth weight babies
	• time consuming, unpleasant, and costly
	• causes unnecessary anxiety

Effect of recommendation on feelings, beliefs, values of self and family:

Physician-patient partnership decision   Date _____

Follow-up plan:

14.3   SCREENING FOR BACTERIA IN THE URINE DURING PREGNANCY

Since the early 1950s the idea that all pregnant women need urine tests to detect infection, even if they have no symptoms, has been promoted. The rationale for the test is that as pregnancy advances, pressure from the growing baby prevents urine from flowing freely from the kidney to the bladder, and the reduction of urine flow could lead to kidney infections that otherwise would not occur. Infection in the kidneys can be serious for both mother and baby. Testing the urine at 16 weeks of pregnancy and treating the mother with antibiotics, if necessary, should prevent serious problems from developing.

Evidence

Studies have shown that women found to have bacteria in their urine at 12 to 16 weeks of pregnancy have a 13% chance of developing a serious kidney infection later in the pregnancy. Only 0.4% of women with sterile urine on testing at 16 weeks go on to develop an infection.[1] Before antibiotics were available, women who suffered from kidney infections during pregnancy were more likely to have babies with low birth weight, and there was a higher risk of the baby dying during or shortly after birth.[2] The presence of bacteria in the urine at 16 weeks has been associated with an increased chance of infant death which is 2.4 times that of women with sterile urine. Bacteria in the urine also leads to reduced growth of the baby during the pregnancy.[3]

A meta-analysis found that women with bacteria in their urine had a 54% higher rate of preterm labor than women whose urine was not infected.[4] Another study found that 40% of women with infected urine developed a uterine infection after the baby was born.[5] No study has found that a urinary tract infection during pregnancy causes permanent kidney damage or high blood pressure later in life.

Method of Bacteria Detection

A urine "dipslide" test for bacteria between 12 and 16 weeks is the most accurate test. If the test indicates bacteria are present, a second test should be performed. If the second test is positive, a sterile urine sample should be obtained and the bacteria grown (cultured) for identification, so that specific treatment can be given. This procedure will detect 80% of women with bacteria in their urine.[6] It has been shown that further monthly testing provides little additional benefit.

Four studies have found that acute kidney infections were prevented in 20 to 30% of women who had bacteria detected by the urine dipslide procedure and had the bacteria eliminated by antibiotic treatment early in the pregnancy.[1,6–8] Although some investigators have questioned the cost-effectiveness of the test, most agree that a single urine dipslide test for bacteria between 12 and 16 weeks of pregnancy is appropriate.[9]

RECOMMENDATION

All pregnant women should undergo a single urine dipslide test for bacteria between 12 and 16 weeks of pregnancy. If the test is positive, it should be repeated and urine for culture should be obtained. All women with bacteria in their urine should be treated with appropriate antibiotics and have follow-up tests to ensure that the infection is gone. (It should be noted that few physicians use the dipslide method of testing. Some use the readily available dipstick test, checking for leukocytes and nitrites. This is not a good screening test. Most do a urine culture directly.)

OTHER RECOMMENDATIONS

Both the U.S. Preventive Services Task Force and the Canadian Task Force on the Periodic Health Examination recommend screening for asymptomatic bacteriuria in pregnancy. The Canadian Task Force gives this screening test an "A" recommendation.

REFERENCES

1.   Kinkaid-Smith P, Buller M. Bacteriuria in pregnancy. Lancet 1965;i:395–399.

2.   Norden W, Kass EH. Bacteriuria of pregnancy-a critical appraisal. Ann Rev Med 1968;19:431–470.

3.   McGrady GA, Daling JR, Peterson DR. Maternal urinary tract infection and adverse fetal outcomes. Am J Epidemiol 1985;121:377–381.

4.   Romero R, Oyarzun E, Mazor M, et al. Meta-analysis of the relationship between asymptomatic bacteriuria and preterm delivery/low birth weight. Obstet Gynecol 1989;73:576–582.

5.   Monif GRG. Intrapartum bacteriuria and postpartum endometritis. Obstet Gynecol 1991;78:245–248.

6.   Stenqvist K, Dahlen-Nillson I, Lidin-Janson G, et al. Bacteriuria in pregnancy: 1. Frequency and risk of acquisition. Am J Epidemiol 1989;129:372–379.

7.   Patterson TF, Andriole VT. Bacteriuria in pregnancy. Infect Dis Clin North Am 1987;1:807–822.

8.   Little PJ. The incidence of urinary tract infection in 5000 pregnant women. Lancet 1966;ii(470):925–928.

9.   Campbell-Brown M, McFadyen IR, Seal DV, et al. Is screening for bacteriuria in pregnancy worthwhile? Br Med J Clin Res Ed 1987;294:1579–1582.

Physician-Patient Partnership Paper

Patient_____

Chart I.D. _____

Physician _____

The Question:
Should I have my urine tested for bacteria between 12 and 16 weeks of pregnancy?

Information about current health, past health, and family health relevant to the question:

Medical Evidence:
Recommendation: Every pregnant woman should be tested for bacteriuria between 12 and 16 weeks of pregnancy.

Advantages
- early detection and treatment prevents kidney infection
- reduces risk of low birth weight and premature labor
- reduces perinatal mortality

Disadvantages
- undergoing urine test
- cost-effectiveness debated

Effect of recommendation on feelings, beliefs, values of self and family:

Physician-patient partnership decision   Date _____

Follow-up plan:

14.4   HOME UTERINE ACTIVITY MONITORING TO PREVENT PRETERM BIRTH

A number of studies have suggested that between the 26th and 36th weeks of pregnancy women should count the movements of their baby at set times each day. The counting of fetal movements will detect changes in activity which could predict problems with the baby that might lead to preterm birth. Detection of distress in the baby could allow the early use of drugs to stop premature labor. Six percent of all births occur before 36 weeks of pregnancy. These early births account for a high percentage of perinatal deaths, as well as nervous system damage to surviving babies.

The recommended method of uterine-activity monitoring requires that the woman count the baby's movements for 5 to 20 minutes, 2 to 4 times daily. If the movements change pattern, in the following days, the woman should rest by lying on her side, drink extra amounts of fluid, and monitor more frequently. If the movements do not return to normal, hospitalization for further management is suggested.

Evidence of Benefit

There have been four randomized controlled trials to measure the benefit of fetal movement monitoring to prevent early labor and premature delivery. Each study involved a small number of women and was flawed in design. One of the main problems with the study design was that the women not using home uterine monitoring received much less medical contact and attention than the women who were reporting daily. Two of the four studies found that the women participating in home fetal monitoring had the same number of preterm births as those not participating.[1,2] In the other two trials, there were slightly fewer preterm births in the monitoring group.[3,4] All the studies found that the procedure was both demanding and expensive, costing between $7,000 and $12,000 per pregnancy. The costs include physician visits and personnel employed for the mother to report to daily. More significant costs would incur with in-hospital management with seemingly little or no benefit and much parental anxiety.

RECOMMENDATION

Home uterine-activity monitoring (H.U.A.M.) is not recommended for normal pregnancy because of cost and the lack of demonstrated benefit. For a woman with a past history of premature birth, or a high-risk pregnancy, the recommendation is not clear and should be individualized.

RECOMMENDATION OF OTHERS

The Canadian Task Force on the Periodic Health Examination and the U.S. Preventive Services Task Force both give H.U.A.M. a "D" recommendation for normal pregnancy and a "C" recommendation for pregnancies considered at high risk for premature births.

REFERENCES

1.   Morrison JC, Martin JN Jr, Martin RW, et al. A program of uterine activity monitoring and its effect on neonatal morbidity. J Perinatol 1988;8:228–231.

2.   Iams JD, Johnson FF, O'Shaughnessy RW, et al. A prospective random trial of home uterine activity monitoring in pregnancies at increased risk of preterm labor. Am J Obstet Gynecol 1987;157:638–643.

3.   Dyson DC, Crites YM, Ray DA, et al. Prevention of preterm birth in high risk patients: The role of education and provider contact versus home uterine monitoring. Am J Obstet Gynecol 1991;164:756–762.

4.   Mou SM, Sunderji SG, Gall S, et al. Multicenter randomized clinical trial of home uterine activity monitoring for detection of preterm labor. Am J Obstet Gynecol 1991;165:858–866.

Physician-Patient Partnership Paper

Patient _____

Chart I.D. _____

Physician _____

The Question:
Should I monitor my baby's movements between 26 and 36 weeks of pregnancy?

Information about current health, past health, and family health relevant to the question:

Medical Evidence:
Recommendation: In normal pregnancy monitoring is not recommended. In high-risk pregnancy there is no clear benefit but the use should be discussed.

Advantages
- very close monitoring of the pregnancy
- may have benefit in pregnancy at risk for premature labor

Disadvantages
- no good evidence of benefit in normal pregnancy
- demanding of women's time
- cost
- anxiety provoking

Effect of recommendation on feelings, beliefs, values of self and family:

Physician-patient partnership decision   Date _____

Follow-up plan:

14.5   CONTINUOUS ELECTRONIC MONITORING OF THE BABY DURING LABOR

The usual method to monitor a baby's heartbeat during labor is to have a doctor, midwife, or nurse listen at intervals with a stethoscope. Electronic monitoring is carried out through an abdominal microphone, or an electrode attached to the baby's scalp through the mother's cervix. The baby's heartbeat can be continuously monitored and recorded. During a normal labor, the baby's heart rate varies considerably. During strong contractions of the uterus, the pressure on a baby's head causes the heart rate to drop. When the pressure is relieved between contractions, the heart rate tends to rise. Physicians, nurses, midwives, and parents may become anxious as they watch and hear these variations and attempt to interpret them. Certain patterns of fetal heart rate may indicate a drop in the baby's oxygen level which could lead to brain damage. However, the connection between the heart rate and oxygen levels in a baby's bloodstream has been very difficult to demonstrate.

Evidence of Benefit

Although eight studies have been carried out comparing electronic fetal monitoring during labor with the traditional occasional listening, only two of these trials are large enough to provide meaningful conclusions.[1–8] The studies used the APGAR score of the newborn at 5 minutes after birth as the outcome measure. Some studies also followed the babies' health for up to 1 year.

Four reviews of the literature published about continuous electronic fetal monitoring have drawn similar conclusions.[6–9] There is no benefit in terms of the overall health of the baby when measured up to 1 year after birth. The reviews found a higher rate of cesarean section in continuously electronically monitored mothers. There was a higher rate of seizures in unmonitored newborns. Mothers whose babies had continuous scalp clip monitoring had a higher rate of infection after the baby was born than mothers who had conventional monitoring.[9]

Evidence of Benefit in High Risk Labor

Trials have been conducted in which mothers, considered by accepted criteria to have high-risk pregnancies, were randomly allocated to receive electronic monitoring or the traditional listening approach. Although there was no difference found between babies whose mothers' labor was monitored either way, mothers who had continuous electronic monitoring underwent significantly more cesarean sections.[1–5] These trials involved numbers too small to detect a minor benefit that might have occurred in either group.

Evidence of Benefit in Normal Labor

The largest well-designed study of electronic fetal monitoring of normal pregnancies involved 12,964 women in Dublin, Ireland. The study found women who had electronic fetal monitoring had a significantly higher rate of cesarean sections when compared to those receiving traditional monitoring. Traditionally monitored babies had more seizures at birth. Follow-up of babies who suffered seizures at birth and babies that did not have seizures found no difference between the two groups after 1 year.[7]

RECOMMENDATION

The evidence does not support the use of continuous electronic fetal monitoring in normal pregnancy and normal labor. There is no evidence of significant benefit to the baby, and there is evidence of a significantly higher cesarean section rate. For women whose pregnancy is considered high risk, there is little evidence of benefit from continuous electronic monitoring. Continuous electronic monitoring may be beneficial if conventional monitoring is difficult.

RECOMMENDATION OF OTHERS

The Canadian Task Force on the Periodic Health Examination gives continuous electronic fetal monitoring a "D" recommendation for normal low-risk pregnancies. The Canadian Task Force gives use of continuous electronic monitoring in high-risk pregnancies a "C" recommendation. The U.S. Preventive Services Task Force has not made a recommendation on this subject.

REFERENCES

1.   Renou P, Chang A, Anderson I, et al. Controlled trial of fetal intensive care. Am J Obstet Gynecol 1976;126:470–476.

2.   Havercamp AD, Thompson HE, McFee JG, et al. The evaluation of continuous fetal heart rate monitoring in high-risk pregnancy. Am J Obstet Gynecol 1976;125:310–320.

3.   Havercamp AD, Orleans M, Langendoerfer S, et al. A controlled trial of the differential effects of intrapartum fetal monitoring. Am J Obstet Gynecol 1979;134:399–412.

4.   Luthy DA, Shy KK, vanBell G, et al. A randomized trial of electronic fetal monitoring in preterm labor. Obstet Gynecol 1987;69:687–695.

5.   Kelso IM, Parsons RJ, Lawrence GF, et al. An assessment of continuous fetal heart rate monitoring in labor. Am J Obstet Gynecol 1978;131:526–532.

6.   Wood C, Renou P, Oates J, et al. A controlled trial of fetal heart rate monitoring in a low risk obstetric population. Am J Obstet Gynecol 1981;141:527–534.

7.   MacDonald D, Grant A, Sheridan-Pereira M, et al. The Dublin randomized controlled trial of intrapartum fetal heart rate monitoring. Am J Obstet Gynecol 1985;152:524–539.

8.   Leveno KJ, Cuningham FG, Nelson S, et al. A prospective comparison of selective and universal electronic fetal monitoring in 34,995 pregnancies. N Engl J Med 1986;315:615–619.

9.   Grant AM. EFM vs intermittent auscultation in labor: EFM + scalp sampling vs intermittent auscultation in labor: Liberal vs restrictive use of EFM in labor (all labor); liberal vs restrictive use in labor (low risk labor); In pregnancy and childbirth module (eds. Enkin MW, Keirse MJNC, Renfrew MJ, Neilson JP. "Cochrane Data Base of Systematic Reviews" review no.s 03884, 03297, 03885, 03886 First two released May 4, 1994 second two released April 8, 1994.

Physician-Patient Partnership Paper

Patient _____

Chart I.D. _____

Physician _____

The Question: Should my baby's heart rate be electronically monitored during labor?

Information about current health, past health, and family health relevant to the question:

Medical Evidence:

Recommendation: Continuous electronic fetal monitoring during normal labor is not recommended. In high-risk or difficult situations it may be considered.

Advantages
- more accurate monitoring of heart beat
- provides record of labor
- lower rate of seizures in newborn

Disadvantages
- results in higher C-section rate
- creates anxiety
- no proven benefit
- increased rate of maternal postpartum infection with scalp electrode

Effect of recommendation on feelings, beliefs, values of self and family:

Physician-patient partnership decision   Date _____

Follow-up plan:

Physician-Patient Partnership Papers for Newborns and Young Children

15.1 THE WELL-BABY EXAMINATION IN THE FIRST TWO YEARS

Several studies have attempted to determine how many doctor visits a healthy baby should have during the first two years. The purpose of these visits is to immunize the baby, as well as to detect any congenital or other illness. Studies have shown that immunization and appropriate disease prevention can be achieved with one visit during the first month of life, followed by visits at 2, 4, 6, 12 to 15, and 18 months of age. Any acute illness during this time will require extra visits.[1]

No studies have shown any benefit from more frequent visits if the child is normal and healthy. During the past few years new mothers have been leaving hospital within 12 hours of delivery resulting in extra visits to the doctor for help with breast-feeding, investigation of jaundice, or other problems that may concern new parents and require physician support, especially for first-time mothers.

What Should be Checked on a Well-Baby Visit to the Doctor?

Parents' Concerns

Caring for a newborn, especially one's first, is difficult. Since many people have raised children, advice is readily available even though some of it may not be particularly helpful. The well-baby visit provides an opportunity to answer parents' questions and to provide sound advice about health and safety measures.

Child Safety and Injury Prevention

The most common cause of all deaths in babies under 1 is accidents. In the developed countries, injuries cause at least four times as many deaths in this age group as disease.

The most common preventable cause of death is motor vehicle accidents. The most effective preventive step is to always properly buckle the baby into an approved infant car seat when the car is in motion. Safer driving conditions, improvement of roads, and the enforcement of traffic laws will all contribute to improving this preventable loss of life.[2]

Drowning is the second most common preventable cause of death. A reduction of fatalities can only be achieved if infants are never left unsupervised in or near water.

The third most frequent cause of death from injuries is burns or scalds usually resulting from placing the baby in a scalding bath or from spilling hot water from a stove. All parents should check the thermostat on their hot water heater, ensuring that it is at or below 120°F (54°C). Supervision around stoves or any heat source is essential to prevent tragedy.

Choking on small objects like coins, peanuts or similar sized objects, and older sibling's toys is another preventable injury.

Falls from change tables, furniture, infant walkers, and beds can be prevented by careful supervision. A number of excellent booklets providing helpful suggestions about preventing injuries in babies and children can be obtained from a physician or the Public Health Department.

Older children and pets can also be a source of danger.

Problems with Growth and Development

During each well-baby visit to the doctor, a baby's height, weight, and head circumference should be measured and the results recorded on a growth curve chart. The normal expectation is that, although a baby may be above or below average on all measurements, growth will be steady and keep the same pace over time as other babies of the same height or weight. Development also occurs in an expected pattern. If, over several visits, there is deviation from this expected pattern, investigation may be warranted.

Sleep Problems

Night-time awakening and crying after the baby has outgrown night-time feeding requirements occurs in about 20% of babies. If this becomes a cause of worry or concern for the parents, they should seek advice and assistance from their physician on well-baby visits.[3]

Hearing

Serious hearing problems occur in about 1 in 2000 newborns. Deafness should be detected as early as possible, preferably before the child reaches 1 year of age. Often the parents or grandparents are the first to notice that the baby does not respond to loud noises as expected. If a hearing problem is suspected, a simple test which measures a baby's brain responses to noise provides a definitive answer. If a hearing problem is detected, steps can be taken to make a difference in a hearing-impaired child's future functioning.[4]

Amblyopia (crossed eyes)

It is not uncommon for small babies to appear to have crossed or wandering eyes. If an eye is permanently crossed, it should be repaired early to prevent blindness. A simple test a doctor or parent can perform to detect amblyopia is to determine if light from a stationary source is reflected at exactly the same point on both of a baby's pupils. A difference indicates a problem that needs to be dealt with before 1 year of age.[5]

Hip Dislocation

Some babies are born with a dislocated hip, or a hip joint that allows dislocation. Detection of this problem in the first few weeks of life leads to relatively simple treatment that prevents long-term problems. The physician should carry out a test by manipulating a baby's hips at each well-baby visit until a baby is walking.[6]

Tumors of Childhood

These tumors, chiefly renal, adrenal, and retinal, are looked for at every visit.

RECOMMENDATION

Well-baby visits are important for all babies. A physician performs appropriate immunization and looks for problems which, when detected and treated early, reduce or prevent future problems. Six well-baby visits in the first 2 years of life for immunization, discussions about safety, sleep, nutrition, and parenting, and detection of hearing problems, crossed eyes, hip dislocation, and growth and development problems should help a baby achieve its optimum potential.

RECOMMENDATIONS OF OTHERS

The above recommendations are based on the evidence of the Canadian Task Force on the Periodic Health Examination. The U.S. Task Force on the Delivery of Preventive Services generally agrees with these recommendations.

REFERENCES

1. Canadian Task Force on the Periodic Health Examination. The periodic health examination, 1990 update: 4. Well-baby care in the first two years of life. Can Med Assoc J 1990;143(9):867–872.

2. Kelly B, Sein C, McCarthy PL. Safety education in a pediatric primary care setting. Pediatrics 1987; 79:818–824.

3. Rickert VI, Johnson CM. Reducing nocturnal awakening and crying in infants and young children: A comparison between scheduled awakenings and systematic ignoring. Pediatrics 1988;81:203–212.

4. Early identification of hearing impairment in infants and young children. NIH Consensus Statement 1993;11(1):1–24.

5. Lang J. The optimum time for surgical alignment in congenital esotropia. J Pediatr Ophthalmol Strabismus 1984;21:74–75.

6. Dunn PM, Evans RE, Thearle MJ, et al. Congenital dislocation of the hip: early and late diagnosis and management compared. Arch Dis Child 1985;60:407–411.

Physician-Patient Partnership Paper

Patient_____

Chart I.D. _____

Physician _____

The Question: How many visits to the physician should my healthy baby have in the first two years of life? What should be assessed at these visits?

Information about current health, past health, and family health relevant to the question:

Medical Evidence:

Recommendation: There should be a minimum of 6 well-baby visits in the first 2 years. The following should be assessed: immunization, accident prevention, sleeping problems, hearing problems, crossed eyes, hip dislocation, and growth and development.

Advantages
- provides recommended immunization program
- answers parents' questions
- discussion about injury prevention
- discussion about sleep problems
- early detection of deafness with better outcome
- early detection of crossed eyes with better outcome
- early detection of hip dislocation with better outcome
- detecting problems with growth and development
- early detection of tumors

Disadvantages
- risk of immunization reactions (serious reactions about 1/2,000,000)
- six visits too infrequent
- vigorous hip testing may damage joint

Effect of recommendation on feelings, beliefs, values of self and family:

Physician-patient partnership decision   Date _____

Follow-up plan:

15.2 BREAST-FEEDING

Breast-Feeding and Immunity

There are many studies that demonstrate that when clean water and sanitation are not available, as in many developing countries, breast-fed babies have lower rates of infections than bottle-fed babies. Until recently, the benefit of breast-feeding babies in the developed countries, where the risk of infection from the environment is low, was not as apparent. Studies done in the United Kingdom have found benefits to breast-feeding all babies.[1] This study found that only 4% of breast-fed infants suffered a gastrointestinal infection in the first 2 years of life compared to 15% of formula-fed babies. Twenty-six percent of breast-fed infants had at least one cold in the first year of life compared to 37% of formula-fed infants. Even though breast-feeding is often stopped when a baby is 4 to 6 months old, the benefits last for the first 2 years of life. Another study found that 4 months of breast-feeding reduced the risk of acquiring an ear infection during the first year of life by 26%.[2] Breast-feeding babies reduces infection rates by enhancing their immunity to infection.

Breast-Feeding and Allergy Reduction

Several studies have demonstrated that restricting a mother's diet during pregnancy and breast-feeding may reduce the risk of the baby developing allergies. All of the studies have been carried out on women who themselves had major allergy problems. These studies have some flaws which make it difficult to be sure how much the diet restriction or the breast-feeding really contributed.[3] No studies have shown a reduction in allergies in babies who were breast-fed by mothers who did not suffer from allergies or who came from families where there were no allergy sufferers.

Breast-Feeding and Diabetes Prevention

During the past decade a new understanding of the mechanisms by which the body develops diabetes has led to a theory that breast-feeding may reduce the risk of onset of Type I diabetes in children. In Type I diabetes (childhood onset), insulin-producing cells in the pancreas are destroyed by an immune reaction. The body can no longer produce insulin and these persons, usually children or adults under 30, must take insulin injections to control their bodies' use of sugar. One theory of prevention is that breast milk reduces the risk of developing antibodies to the insulin-producing cells.[4] Several large studies comparing children with Type I diabetes to those without found diabetes was less common in those who were breast-fed.[5] It is not possible to do a study that would prove this cause-and-effect relationship, but the theoretical suggestion and the studies suggest a benefit from breast-feeding.

Breast-Feeding and Growth and Development of Babies

There is only one study that properly measured and compared growth rates of breast- and formula-fed babies. Formula-fed babies after 18 months were found to be significantly heavier than breast-fed infants. A debate continues as to whether this finding suggests an increased incidence of adult obesity for the formula-fed. No follow-up studies have been done, adding to confusion surrounding this finding.

RECOMMENDATION

There is evidence that breast-feeding babies for at least 4 to 6 months reduces gastrointestinal, ear, and upper respiratory infections during the first 2 years of life. There is some evidence that a combination of pre- and post-term diet and breast-feeding may reduce the risk of allergies in babies born to mothers with serious allergy problems. There is suggestive evidence that breast-feeding may protect infants or children from developing Type I diabetes. Breast-feeding is recommended as the preferred method of feeding babies, whenever it is feasible.

RECOMMENDATION OF OTHERS

The Canadian Task Force on the Periodic Health Examination gives breast feeding an "A" recommendation, as does the U.S. Preventive Services Task Force. The World Health Organization and UNESCO have developed guidelines promoting breast feeding as the preferred method of feeding all babies. Many other agencies and groups around the world are strongly supportive of this recommendation.

REFERENCES

1. Howie PW, Forsyth JS, Oston SA, et al. Protective effect of breast-feeding against infection. BMJ 1990;300:11–16.

2. Duncan B, Ey J, Holberg CJ, et al. Exclusive breast-feeding for at least four months protects against otitis media. Pediatrics 1993;91:867–872.

3. Kramer MS: Does breast-feeding help protect against atopic disease? Biology, methodology and a golden jubilee of controversy. J Paediatr 1988;112:181–190.

4. Karjalainen J, Martin JM, Knip M, et al. A bovine albumin peptide as a possible trigger of insulin dependent diabetes mellitus. N Engl J Med 1992;327:302–307.

5. Kostraba JN, Cruickshanks KJ, Lawler-Heavner J, et al. Early exposure to cows' milk and solid foods in infancy, genetic predisposition, and risk of IDDM. Diabetes 1993;42:288–295.

Physician-Patient Partnership Paper

Patient_____

Chart I.D. _____

Physician _____

The Question: Should I breast feed my baby?

Information about current health, past health, and family health relevant to the question:

Medical Evidence:

Recommendation: Breast feeding is recommended for all babies for at least 4 to 6 months.

Advantages
- reduced number and severity of gastrointestinal infections, acute and chronic ear infections, and common colds (first 2 years)
- may reduce the risk of allergies in babies whose mother or family has severe allergies
- may reduce the risk of developing diabetes
- no $ cost compared to formula
- no risk of preparation errors or contamination

Disadvantages
- limits mother's absence from baby
- unknown volume of milk intake which can lead to parental anxiety
- problems with nipples or breast engorgement
- may require dietary change for mother
- requires education and support particularly with the first baby
- limits father's role in baby care

Effect of recommendation on feelings, beliefs, values of self and family:

Physician-patient partnership decision   Date _____

Follow-up plan:

15.3   Colds and Sore Throats in Children

Colds and sore throats in children are common health problems. Most babies are protected from colds by their mother's antibodies during their first 3 or 4 months of life. A child averages two colds per year until he/she enters school or join a play group. Children may experience as many as five or six colds per year in their first year or two of exposure to other children.[1]

More than 2000 viruses cause the common cold. There is no effective vaccine. Viruses do not respond to treatment with antibiotics but are controlled by the body's immune system. Most colds run a course of 10 days. Drugs or other measures may relieve some of the symptoms, but will not alter the course of the body's reaction to the virus. Many of the remedies purchased over the counter at a drug store for symptom relief have little benefit and have side effects which are of concern.[2]

The Cold

A viral upper respiratory tract infection (URI) usually begins with nasal obstruction with clear mucus, and a low grade fever around 38°C (100.4°F) orally (rectal temperatures are one degree higher, axillary temperatures one degree lower). Within the first 3 days the fever disappears and the nasal discharge increases to large quantities of green mucus that almost continually block the nasal passage. By day 6 the nasal discharge becomes less copious and becomes sticky and yellow and slowly dries up by day 8 to 10. These symptoms, especially during days 3 to 7, are often accompanied by a cough caused by the discharge from the nose running down the back of the throat, causing an irritation, and producing a minimally productive cough.[1]

The many remedies for the common cold may help to reduce symptoms related to nasal congestion and throat irritation, but may also cause thickened mucous secretions making the person more prone to bacterial infections. No studies have found a drug that significantly alters the cold's natural history.[3] Large quantities of fluids consumed during the course of a cold tend to thin the mucus, allowing it to be more easily cleared. Acetaminophen can be used in the early stages of a cold to relieve fever.

The Sore Throat

If a child's principal complaint is a sore throat, there are several signs suggesting that a bacteria rather than a virus may be the cause of the infection. Streptococcus is one of the common bacteria. It causes a throat infection or "strep" throat. There are several different types of streptococcal bacteria, one of which has been linked to causing rheumatic fever. If this particular "strep" is present, the use of penicillin for 10 days is effective in preventing rheumatic heart disease. Rheumatic heart disease is rare under 2 to 3 years of age and is generally decreasing in incidence.

A recent review of sore throats in adults and children found that 35% of children have a streptococcal infection in their throat when it is sore.[3] This review found that a temperature greater than 38°C orally, tender glands in the neck at the front below the jaw bone, and white spots in the back of the throat or on the tonsils indicate it is likely that strep infection is present, and that an antibiotic should be prescribed. If one or two of these findings is present in the absence of a cough, a throat swab, for strep screen only, should be done. The decision to treat or not should be based on the swab results. Up to 70% of these individuals do not have a bacterial infection and will not benefit from antibiotics. If a person complains of a sore throat but does not have a fever, lymph nodes, or white spots in the throat, a bacterial infection is unlikely. The viral infection should clear without treatment: no throat swab or visit to a physician is necessary.

When a person suffering from a common cold develops any of the above signs, especially a high fever late in the course of a cold, then the possibility of a bacterial infection added to the viral infection should be considered and medical assessment should be sought. Small children may develop ear infections late in the course of a cold.

In adolescents, similar signs may be brought on by infectious mononucleosis which also produces fever, swollen glands in the neck, and exudate.

RECOMMENDATION

Children should have the progress of any upper respiratory tract infection monitored on the basis of the natural history of the common cold. If the cold follows the expected course, increased fluid consumption may be of value. If the progress deviates from what is expected, especially if the fever is greater than 38°C, medical advice should be sought. If the child has no cough but complains of a sore throat, has a fever greater than 38°C, tender glands in the neck, and white spots on the back or side of the throat, it is likely that he/she has a strep infection and would benefit from antibiotics. If there are one or two findings but no cough, a throat swab should be done and the results obtained before antibiotics are given. If the only complaint is a sore throat without tender glands, spots in the throat, and fever, no treatment is indicated.

REFERENCES

1.   Feldman W, Rosser WW, McGrath P. Primary Medical Care of Children and Adolescents. New York: Oxford University Press, 1987:9.

2.   Brazie DB, Dennie FW, Dillon HC, et al. Difficult management problems in children with streptococcal pharyngitis. Pediatr Infect Dis 1985;4:10–13.

3.   McIsacc WJ, Goel V, Slaughter PM, et al. Reconsidering sore throats, Part 2: Alternative approaches and practical office tool. Can Fam Physician 1997;3:495–500.

Physician-Patient Partnership Paper

Patient_____

Chart I.D. _____

Physician _____

The Question: Should my child get antibiotics to help him/her get over a cold?

Information about current health, past health, and family health relevant to the question:

Medical Evidence:

Recommendation: If the cold follows its natural course, no antibiotics will be helpful. If there is a sore throat with no cough, but fever greater than 38°C, tender neck glands, and white spots in the throat, antibiotics are indicated.

Advantages	*Disadvantages*
• treat bacterial infections effectively	• do cause allergic and other drug reactions
• may inhibit development of rheumatic heart disease	• have no effect on viral infections
	• unnecessary use increases bacterial resistance to antibiotics in the community
	• cost

Effect of recommendation on feelings, beliefs, values of self and family:

Physician-patient partnership decision   Date _____

Follow-up plan:

15.4   Ear Infections in Children

Ear infections in children under the age of 5 are a common problem. They tend to occur when a child is first exposed to other children in play groups or day care or to older siblings who bring home an infection. Most children suffer at least one ear infection before they reach the age of 5 and some children have had 5 or 6 ear infections by their second or third year of life.[1] It has been estimated that in the US at least $1 billion is spent annually on antibiotics, and $3.5 billion on other drugs, physicians, and surgery for ear infections.

About 70% of ear infections follow a cold or nasal congestion which causes swelling and obstruction of the eustachian tubes that connect the back of the nose to the middle ear. Children under 5 are more likely to have swelling and obstruction of the eustachian tubes because the openings are very small. As the child grows, the tubes enlarge and the likelihood of blockage decreases.

An open eustachian tube allows fluid from behind the eardrum to discharge into the back of the nose. With closure of the tube, fluid accumulates in the middle ear. Twenty percent of infections in this situation are caused by viruses, 20 to 30% are mixed bacterial and viral, and 50% are caused by bacteria alone. Hearing can be temporarily affected in 25 to 30% of children as the pressure from the fluid reduces the ability of the eardrum to vibrate.

When the canal is blocked and infection is present in the middle ear, the pressure may cause the eardrum to burst. This allows the pus to drain and equalizes the pressure, relieving the pain and fever. The same relief can result if the pressure pushes the eustachian tube open. One might expect that breaking or rupturing the ear drum would cause damage and permanently affect hearing, but this does not seem to be the case.[2]

Treatment

Treatment of acute otitis media (infection of the middle ear) is based on the premise that the best way to treat it is to kill the bacteria with antibiotics. There is growing evidence that because of the way the middle ear functions, awaiting the opening of the blocked eustachian tube may offer a better alternative.

In the US and Canada, ear infections are treated with a 10-day course of antibiotics from the time they are discovered. In the United Kingdom, 5 days of antibiotics are traditionally used to manage middle ear infections. In Holland, children with middle ear infections are less likely to be brought to a physician, but when they are, children are given medication for fever and pain (acetaminophen every 4 hours according to age and weight) and advised to return to the physician in 24 hours if less than 2 years old, or 72 hours if older than 2 years, if the fever, pain or other symptoms have not resolved. Children who appear to be very ill are treated with antibiotics.[3]

In a Dutch study, only 10% of children returned for antibiotics (15% were given antibiotics when they were first seen by their physician). The preliminary outcome findings suggest that there are no differences in complication rates for the three groups.

The explanation for the reduced use of antibiotics is related to middle ear functioning. It seems most blocked eustachian tubes open within 24 to 72 hours. Only if the eustachian tube remains blocked or the infection spreads does the child need antibiotics. The Dutch findings suggest that 75% of ear infections clear on their own and about 25% of children need antibiotics.[4]

A large, four-country study, soon to be reported in the medical literature, has compared the three approaches to managing ear infection. The children are being monitored for 6 months after the infection to determine if there are any differences in hearing or other complications.

Reducing the use of antibiotics for this common problem has been shown to reduce the growing number of strains of bacteria resistant to antibiotics. This is an issue of growing importance in North America.[5]

RECOMMENDATION

For a child with fever and other symptoms of an acute middle ear infection, there is growing evidence that treating with acetaminophen and following the course of the illness for 24 hours if the child is under 2 years old, or 72 hours if over 2, is the most appropriate approach. Antibiotics may be needed immediately by the 15% of children who are very ill. If more serious symptoms develop, or the fever, pain and other symptoms do not resolve within the recommended time frame, antibiotics use should be considered. This approach to treatment of ear infections is very different from the usual North American management. Both the physician and parents must understand the approach and be comfortable with it before implementation.

RECOMMENDATION OF OTHERS

There are at present no recommendations in North America that suggest any change from the current approach of 10 days of antibiotics for acute middle ear infections.

REFERENCES

1.   Bluestone CD. Otitis media in children. To treat or not to treat. N Engl J Med 1982;306:1399–1404.

2.   Northern JL, Downs MP. Hearing in Children. Baltimore: Williams and Wilkins, 1974:97.

3.   Delmar C, Glaz P, Hayem M. Are antibiotics indicated in the initial treatment for children with acute otitis media? A meta-analysis. BMJ 1997;314:1526–1530.

4.   Froom S, Culpepper L, Greb P, et al. Diagnosis and antibiotic treatment of acute otitis media. A Report from International Primary Care Network. BMJ 1990;300:582–586.

5.   von Buchen FL, Dunk JHM, van't Hof MA. Therapy of acute otitis media: myringotomy, antibiotics or neither? A double-blind study in children. Lancet 1981;ii:883–887.

Physician-Patient Partnership Paper

Patient _____

Chart I.D. _____

Physician _____

The Question: Should my child receive antibiotics in the first 24 to 72 hours of ear infection?

Information about current health, past health, and family health relevant to the question:

Medical Evidence:

Recommendation: Treat children who are very ill with antibiotics immediately. Treat all others for fever and pain only and follow up according to age — in 24 hours if under 2 years, and 72 hours if over 2 years. Treat with antibiotics if more serious symptoms develop, or the fever, pain, and other symptoms do not resolve within the time frame.

Advantages	*Disadvantages*
• reduces use of antibiotics	• not the conventional therapy
• reduces complications from antibiotics	• delays onset of therapy for some who would benefit
• less expensive	
• reduces development of resistance to antibiotics	• may prolong illness for some

Effect of recommendation on feelings, beliefs, values of self and family:

Physician-patient partnership decision   Date _____

Follow-up plan:

15.5 IMMUNIZING CHILDREN

Immunizing children against infectious disease has been one of mankind's greatest advances. All children should routinely receive immunization against diphtheria, pertussis (whooping cough), tetanus (lock jaw), polio, measles, mumps, rubella, hemophilia, and hepatitis-B.

Concerns have been raised about the risks of some vaccines. Much of the controversy arose in the UK over pertussis vaccine. Severe or even lethal reactions to vaccines are recorded, but rare. The best way to weigh the risk of reaction is to compare it with the risk of suffering the actual disease. Table 1 addresses this issue for pertussis vaccine and provides overwhelming evidence of benefit from the vaccine. The new acellular pertussis vaccine coming into use has an even lower risk of reaction. The Scandinavian countries have decided that individuals reacting to a vaccine should be compensated by society, since there is societal benefit in having everyone receive the vaccines. Most countries are not so enlightened and compensation for serious reactions to vaccination is left to the courts. This is costly for both the families and the vaccine manufacturers and in some countries has jeopardized the viability of vaccine producers.

RECOMMENDATION

Table 2 outlines the generally recommended immunization schedule. Timing varies from region to region. The program is designed to occur in conjunction with regularly scheduled well-baby visits. The program for hepatitis-B is arbitrary as the best time to give the vaccine has not been determined. The recommendation is currently the same as for mothers positive for antibodies to hepatitis-B.

All of the vaccines in Table 2 are strongly recommended because of the high benefit-to-risk ratio that each vaccine carries. There have been questions about the need for a tetanus booster every 10 years after the initial childhood program. A study in Canada over a 10-year period was unable to find even one case of tetanus in individuals who had received the childhood immunization program.[3] This study suggested that tetanus boosters are likely not necessary after the childhood program. There may be some benefit to having a booster when a wound at high risk for tetanus is incurred, but there is no evidence to support this.

RECOMMENDATIONS OF OTHERS

The Canadian Task Force on the Periodic Health Examination gives an "A" recommendation to the above schedule. Although there are minor variations in timing, most other organizations agree with this outline.

Table 1   Risk of Reaction after Pertussis Vaccine [2]

Problem	Risk from Vaccine	Risk from Disease	Relative Risk Ratio
Seizures	1:1750	1:25–1:250	7–70:1
Shock	1:1750	not known	not known
Brain inflammation	1:110,000	1:1.000–1:4,000	28–110:1
Brain damage	1:310,000	1:2,000–1:8,000	39–155:1
Death	1:1,000,000	1:200–1:1,000	1,000–5,000:1

Table 2   Recommended Vaccine Schedule

Age of Baby/Child	Recommended Vaccine	Need and Age for Booster
Birth	Hep-B	
One Month	Hep-B	
Two Months	DPTP Hem	
Four Months	DPTP Hem	
Six Months	DPTP Hem, Hep-B	
Twelve Months	MMR	MMR (4–6 years)
Eighteen Months	DPTP Hem	DPTP (4–6 years)

REFERENCES

1.   The Canadian Task Force on the Periodic Health Examination. The Canadian Guide to Clinical Preventive Health Care. Ottawa: Minister of Supply and Services, 1994:372–384.

2.   Gold R. Pertussis and pertussis vaccine. Canada Disease Weekly Report 1985;11:8.

3.   Rosser WW, Hutchison BG, McDowell I, Newell C. Use of reminders to increase compliance with tetanus booster vaccination. Can Med Assoc J 1992;146:911–917.

Physician-Patient Partnership Paper

Patient_____

Chart I.D. _____

Physician _____

The Question: Should my child be immunized?

Information about current health, past health, and family health relevant to the question:

Medical Evidence:

Recommendation: The full course of immunization should be received by all.

Advantages
- high level of protection against specific childhood diseases for the individual
- societal protection against epidemics of specific illnesses

Disadvantages
- frequent mild reactions with rare serious reactions

Effect of recommendation on feelings, beliefs, values of self and family:

Physician-patient partnership decision   Date _____

Follow-up plan:

CHAPTER 16

Physician-Patient Partnership Papers for Cardiovascular Disease

16.1 CONTROLLING BLOOD PRESSURE IN PEOPLE UNDER 65

Blood Pressure Measurement

It is estimated that 15% of the adult population has high blood pressure. When having a blood pressure reading taken, one should avoid smoking, or the consumption of caffeinated drinks 30 minutes prior to the blood pressure reading. The reading should be taken in a relaxed atmosphere.

If the diastolic blood pressure is found to be above 90 mm Hg on three separate readings over a period of 3 to 6 months, and measures such as weight reduction and increased exercise have not lowered the pressure to normal, the implementation of drug therapy may be indicated.[1] The beginning of drug therapy may occur sooner if the individual involved has other cardiovascular risk factors such as smoking, diabetes, strong family history of heart disease or stroke, high serum cholesterol, a high alcohol intake, or marked obesity accompanied by a sedentary lifestyle.

Although there is evidence of benefit from treating persons over 21 for diastolic blood pressures greater than 90 mm Hg, there has been some reluctance to initiate drug therapy immediately in the absence of any other risk factors. Once the diastolic blood pressure on three or more readings is greater than 100 mm Hg, then the evidence of benefit increases.[1]

There are no long-term studies that focus on systolic blood pressure. Most physicians treat when the systolic blood pressure is greater than 140 to 160, with a lowered threshold for treating if other risk factors are present.

Although many guidelines and academic groups recommend that evidence of end-organ damage to blood vessels, the heart, kidneys and/or the brain is an indication to begin drug therapy immediately, there is little evidence from several large studies to support this approach.[2–4]

Benefits from Treatment

There have been only short-term trials where lifestyle modification was attempted, and there is no evidence of benefits to lowering the stroke or heart attack rates.[5]

Long-term treatment with drugs lowers the diastolic pressure an average of 4 to 6 mm Hg. A number of studies have demonstrated that lowering blood pressure significantly reduces the number and severity of strokes and, to a lesser extent, the rate of heart attacks.[6,7]

When a number of studies on the benefits of blood pressure lowering were merged (meta-analysis), an average of 5 to 6 mm Hg lowering of the diastolic blood pressure resulted in a 42% reduction in fatal and nonfatal strokes and a 14% reduction in heart attacks.[8] The full benefit of treatment in preventing strokes is observed in as few as 3 years of treatment while the benefit in heart attack reduction requires 5 or more years. For reasons that are not entirely clear, women do not benefit as much as men.[9]

Almost all the long-term treatment studies have been carried out using diuretics and/or beta blockers. In one large trial, 20% of persons had stopped the drugs within 5 years because of minor side effects.[7] There are now a number of antihypertensive drugs available including calcium channel blockers, angiotensin converting enzyme (ACE) inhibitors, and alpha-adrenergic blockers. These drugs have been shown to be as effective as the older drugs and many believe they have fewer side effects.[10,11] Specific patient groups appear to benefit from these drugs,[12,13] but there are no long-term trials demonstrating greater longevity or safety over the older, less expensive drugs.

RECOMMENDATION

All persons between the ages of 21 and 65 should have their blood pressure accurately measured in a medical facility once every 2 or 3 years.[10] If the blood pressure is found on three separate occasions over a 3- to 6-month period to have a diastolic reading greater than 90 mm Hg, lifestyle modification should be attempted prior to consideration of drug therapy. This decision will be influenced by the presence of other cardiovascular risk factors. If the diastolic pressure is greater than 100 mm Hg or there is evidence of damage from elevated blood pressure to the blood vessels in the eye, heart or kidneys, drug therapy should be initiated immediately.[3]

RECOMMENDATION OF OTHERS

The Canadian Task Force on the Periodic Health Examination gives a "B" recommendation to the regular testing of the blood pressure of all adults aged 21 to 65. It gives an "A" recommendation to the treatment of anyone in this age group found to have accurately measured diastolic blood pressure greater than 90 mm Hg on three separate occasions. Most guidelines favor the use of diuretics or beta blockers as the drugs of choice for initiating therapy.

The U.S. Preventive Services Task Force recommends the measurement of blood pressure beginning at the age of 3. It agrees with the other recommendations of the Canadian Task Force.

REFERENCES

1.   Collins R, Peto R, MacMahon S, et al. Blood pressure and coronary heart disease. Part 2. Short term reductions in blood pressure: Overview of randomized drug trials in their epidemiological context. Lancet 1990;335:827–838.

2.   Multiple Risk Factor Intervention Trial Research Group. Multiple risk factor intervention trial: risk factor changes and mortality results. JAMA 1982;248:1465–1477.

3.   Wilhelmsen L, Berglund G, Elmfeldt D, et al. The multifactor primary prevention trial in Goteborg, Sweden. Eur Heart J 1986;7:279–288.

4.   Sirandberg TE, Salomaa UVV, Naukarien VA, et al. Long term mortality after 5 year multifactorial primary prevention of cardiovascular disease in middle-aged men. JAMA 1991;266:1225–1229.

5.   National High Blood Pressure Education Program. The fifth report of the joint national committee on detection, evaluation, and treatment of high blood pressure. Arch Intern Med 1993;153:154–183.

6.   Report by the Management Committee. The Australian therapeutic trial in mild hypertension. Lancet 1980;i:1261–1267.

7.   Medical Research Council Working Party: MRC trial of treatment of mild hypertension: principal results. Br Med J Clin Res Ed 1985;291:97–104.

8.   MacMahon SW, Cutler JA, Furberg CD, et al. The effects of drug treatment for hypertension on morbidity and mortality from cardiovascular disease: review of randomized controlled trials. Prog Cardiovasc Dis 1986;24(3)(Suppl 1):99–118.

9.   The management committee of the Australian National Blood Pressure Study. Prognostic factors in the treatment of mild hypertension. Circulation 1984;69:668–676.

10.   Fletcher AE, Bulpit CJ, Chase DM, et al. Quality of life with three anti-hypertensive treatments: Cilazapril, atenolol, nifedipine. Hypertension 1992;19:499–507.

11.   The treatment of mild hypertension research group. The treatment of mild hypertension study. A randomized, placebo-controlled trial of a nutritional hygienic regimen along with various drug monotherapies. Arch Intern Med 1991;151:1413–1423.

12.   Lewis EJ, Hunsicker LG, Bain RP, et al. The effect of angiotensin-converting-enzyme inhibition on diabetic nephropathy. New Engl J Med 1993;329:1456–1462.

13.   Carruthers SG, Larochelle P, Haynes RB, et al. Report of the Canadian Hypertension Society Consensus Conference. 1. [Introduction] Can Med Assoc J 1993;149:289–293.

Physician-Patient Partnership Paper

Patient_____

Chart I.D. _____

Physician _____

The Question: Should I have my blood pressure checked once every 2 or 3 years? If my blood pressure is high, should it be treated?

Information about current health, past health, and family health relevant to the question:

Medical Evidence:

Recommendation: Every adult between the ages 21 and 65 should have his/her blood pressure checked every 2 or 3 years. If on three readings it is found elevated, or there is target-organ damage, it should be treated.

Advantages	*Disadvantages*
• reduced stroke and heart attack rate	• need for follow-up
• simple inexpensive test	• may require lifestyle change which can be difficult
• treatment may be simple and inexpensive, and may involve lifestyle change only	• drugs may have side effects
	• cost

Effect of recommendation on feelings, beliefs, values of self and family:

Physician-patient partnership decision   Date _____

Follow-up plan:

16.2 CONTROLLING BLOOD PRESSURE IN PEOPLE OVER 65

During the past 20 years there has been a debate over the maximum age at which benefits of blood pressure lowering are realized. American physicians have argued that the benefits of lowering blood pressure, even though demonstrated only to age 65, should be extrapolated to any age. British physicians have argued that those in their 70s and 80s suffer more side effects from drugs and need a higher blood pressure to maintain adequate circulation through less resilient blood vessels. Recent studies have provided a clearer picture of the appropriate way to look for and manage hypertension in the elderly.

Elevated blood pressure in people over 65 is defined as a blood pressure greater than 160 systolic, and greater than 90 diastolic. Ten percent of people over 60 and 20% of people over 80 have elevated blood pressure by this definition.[1]

Prior to having their blood pressure taken, people over 65 must abstain from ingesting caffeine and smoking for 30 minutes. The test should be carried out in as relaxed an atmosphere as possible. If two readings taken within 5 minutes vary by more than 5 mm Hg, they should be repeated on several occasions.

Four large trials have demonstrated significant benefits from keeping the blood pressure of people over 65 within the normal range.[1–5] These studies found up to a 50% reduction in stroke rate and a 33% reduction in heart attacks using diuretics and secondary drugs, as necessary. The reduction of all-cause mortality was less clear. Because none of the trials had enough number of persons over 80, the benefits for this age group is unclear.

RECOMMENDATION

Everyone over the age of 65 years should have their blood pressure assessed annually. If the pressure is found to be greater than 160/90 on three separate occasions, then initiation of drug therapy may be beneficial. Although there is less clear evidence of benefit in those over 80, trials have not found major adverse effects when therapy is initiated in this age group.

RECOMMENDATION OF OTHERS

The Canadian Task Force on the Periodic Health Examination gives the recommendation for annual screening of patients over 65 a "B", on the basis of weakness in the methods of the trials and a lack of clarity on who should be screened and at what frequency. It gives an "A" recommendation to treating persons between the age of 65 and 80 with blood pressure-lowering drugs to maintain blood pressure below 160/90.

The U.S. Preventive Services Task Force recommends all persons over the age of 3 receive regular blood pressure assessments, and states that blood pressure greater than 140/90 should be treated in all age groups.

REFERENCES

1. Amery A, Birkenhager W, Brixko P, et al. Mortality and morbidity results from the European working party on high blood pressure in the elderly trial. Lancet 1985;i:1349–1354.

2. Vogt TM, Ireland CC, Black D, et al. Recruitment of elderly volunteers for multicenter clinical trial: The SHEP pilot study. Controlled Clin Trials 1986;7:118–133.

3. SHEP cooperative research group: Prevention of stroke by antihypertensive drug treatment in older persons with isolated systolic hypertension. JAMA 1991;265:3255–3264.

4. Dahlof B, Lindholm LH, Hansson L, et al. Morbidity and mortality in the Swedish Trial in old patients with hypertension (STOP HYPERTENSION). Lancet 1991;338:1281–1285.

5. MRC Working Party. Medical Research Council trial of treatment of hypertension in older adults: Principle results. BMJ 1992;304:405–412.

Physician-Patient Partnership Paper

Patient_____

Chart I.D. _____

Physician _____

The Question: Should I have my blood pressure checked once a year? If greater than 160/90, should I take treatment for blood pressure control?

Information about current health, past health, and family health relevant to the question:

Medical Evidence:

Recommendation: Annual blood pressure tests for all persons over 65 are recommended. Any person found on three readings with a blood pressure greater than 160/90 should receive treatment.

Advantages	*Disadvantages*
• simple inexpensive test	• inconvenience of test
• treating high blood pressure reduces risk of heart attack and stroke	• blood pressure treatment has side effects and costs

Effect of recommendation on feelings, beliefs, values of self and family:

Physician-patient partnership decision   Date _____

Follow-up plan:

16.3   USING ASA TO PREVENT HEART ATTACK

It is frequently suggested that men and women over age 50 take acetylsalicylic acid (ASA) on a regular basis to prevent heart attacks. One of the effects of ASA is to reduce blood clotting by reducing the stickiness of platelets in the blood. A heart attack is usually caused by a clot forming in a coronary artery, a vessel that supplies blood to heart muscle. The clot blocks the blood flow to the heart muscle, causing some muscle damage. By reducing the ability of the blood to clot, the chance of clots forming in the coronary arteries is reduced. Strokes are also caused by clots blocking blood flow to the brain. However, some strokes result from bleeding into the brain. In this situation, the brain damage will be more severe if the clotting ability of the blood is reduced.

Given the potential benefits of taking ASA, several large trials have been conducted on 20,000 physicians in the U.K., and 52,000 male physicians and 121,700 nurses in the U.S. to determine the effects of taking ASA.[1–5]

In the British trial there were no significant differences in the rate of stroke or heart attack between the groups taking ASA and those not taking the drug.

In the U.S. physicians' trial, half were assigned to receive a single ASA tablet daily while the other half received a placebo. The follow-up was for an average of 5 years. Those receiving the ASA had significantly fewer fatal and nonfatal heart attacks but a higher stroke rate. When the all-cause mortality was analyzed, there was no difference between those receiving ASA and those receiving the placebo. Studies of subgroups found that those over 50 years of age with low cholesterol levels seemed to benefit most, with a lower rate of heart attack.[3]

In the nurses' study, there was a significant reduction in the rate of both fatal and nonfatal heart attacks in those taking between one and six ASA daily, compared to those not taking ASA. When the results of these trials are combined (meta-analysis), the findings suggest a 33% reduction in nonfatal heart attacks in those taking ASA compared to those in the control group. There was no difference in the rate of fatal stroke or heart attack or nonfatal stroke between those taking and not taking the ASA.[6] Analysis using quality-of-life measures found no significant difference between those taking ASA and the control group.[7]

RECOMMENDATION

When overall benefit is assessed, there remains inadequate evidence to support the daily use of ASA in healthy individuals.

RECOMMENDATION OF OTHERS

The Canadian Task Force on the Periodic Health Examination gives the recommendation to take 325 mg of ASA daily to prevent heart attack or stroke a "C" recommendation. The U.S. Preventive Services Task Force is presently reviewing its recommendation.

REFERENCES

1.   Peto R, Grey R, Collins R, et al. Randomized trial of daily aspirin in British male doctors. BMJ 1988;296:313–316.

2.   Steering Committee of the Physician's Health Study Research group: Preliminary report: Findings of the Aspirin component of the ongoing Physicians Health Study. New Engl J Med 1988;318:262–264.

3.   Steering Committee on the Physician's Health Study Research group. Final report on the aspirin component of the ongoing Physicians Health Study. New Engl J Med 1989;321:129–135.

4. Manson JE, Grobbee DE, Stampfer MJ, et al. Aspirin in the primary prevention of angina pectoris in a randomized trial of United States physicians. Am J Med 1990;89:772–776.

5. Manson JE, Stampfer MJ, Colditz GA, et al. A prospective study of aspirin use and primary prevention of cardiovascular disease in women. JAMA 1991;266(4):521–527.

6. Hennekens CH, Peto R, Hutcheson JB, et al. An overview of the British and American Aspirin studies.[letter] New Engl J Med 1988;318:923–924.

7. Jonas S. The Physician Health Study: A neurologist's concern. Arch Neurol 1990;47:1352–1353.

Physician-Patient Partnership Paper

Patient _____

Chart I.D. _____

Physician _____

The Question: Should I take one aspirin daily to prevent heart attack and stroke?

Information about current health, past health, and family health relevant to the question:

Medical Evidence:

Recommendation: Taking one aspirin daily is not recommended as there is no evidence of overall benefit.

Advantages	*Disadvantages*
• may reduce rate of heart attack and thrombotic stroke	• no evidence of all-cause mortality reduction
• simple, inexpensive	• risk of making hemorrhagic stroke worse
	• may aggravate any bleeding
	• may irritate stomach

Effect of recommendation on feelings, beliefs, values of self and family:

Physician-patient partnership decision   Date _____

Follow-up plan:

16.4 Managing Chest Pain

Whenever an individual feels a twinge of chest pain, anxiety rapidly develops because they usually think of a heart attack. Heart attacks are actually the ninth most common cause of chest pain in adults,[1] and they are rare in anyone under age 40. In this section are descriptions of the common causes of chest pain to help you distinguish between them so that you can respond appropriately.

Causes of Chest Pain

A survey of 832 persons presenting with chest pain to their doctors provides a list of the common causes of chest pain:[1]

Angina pectoris

The most common cause of chest pain, angina pectoris, arises from the heart due to narrowing of the blood vessels supplying the heart muscle. When the heart beats faster, the narrowed blood vessels cannot supply enough blood to the heart muscle and the person experiences chest pain. With rest, the heart slows down, the demand for blood decreases, and the pain is relieved. For many people with angina, the onset of pain is predictable. They know walking up a flight of stairs or climbing up a hill will bring on chest pain. Some people experience the pain when they become nervous or upset.

The pain experienced from angina can be identical to that from a heart attack or from esophageal (food tube) pain. It is described as a tightness, or in more severe episodes, a crushing feeling in the center of the chest at or below the nipple line or high in the stomach area. The tightness is usually not sharp but is very uncomfortable. The pain often radiates into the jaw, shoulder, or arm as far as the elbow or even the wrist. The main characteristic of angina is that the pain goes away after 10 minutes of rest. Heart attack pain continues and is not affected by rest or position change; any chest pain of this description lasting more than 15 to 30 minutes should be considered a heart attack until diagnosed otherwise. Most people suffering from angina are over age 50, are familiar with their condition, have drugs (nitroglycerine) that will quickly relieve the pain, and may take drugs that slow the heart rate and reduce the risk of developing anginal pain.

Chest Wall Pain

The second most common cause of chest pain is stretching or pulling on the muscles of the rib cage. The muscles between each rib are quite sensitive since, unlike most muscles in the body, they never rest; they have to move with every breath. Pain from muscle strain in the chest wall may occur anywhere in the chest, but most often it occurs on the front of the chest, either on the left or right upper half, where the muscles from the arms are attached. The pain is sharp, localized and the area is tender when pressed. The pain can be severe and can worsen with breathing or movement.

Pain from the Stomach and Esophagus

The pain-sensitive nerves in the heart are the same nerves sensitive to irritation in the esophagus and upper stomach. Pain from stomach irritation is often described as having a burning quality, but it may be identical to angina pain. Sometimes the pain may be relieved by use of an antacid, but this does not ensure that the heart is not the source of the discomfort. The main distinguishing feature between esophagal pain and heart pain is the sufferer's age. If the person is under 40, the pain is most likely from the stomach or esophagus. This is especially true if large amounts of alcohol have been consumed or gastric irritation (nausea or vomiting) has recently been suffered. If the person is between 40 and 60 and complains of angina-like pain, it should be assumed to come from the heart until proven otherwise. If the sufferer is over 60, the pain is likely cardiac.

Despite years of research, it remains difficult for physicians to accurately distinguish between pain of cardiac origin and gastrointestinal (GI) origin, even with blood tests.[2,3] The result of this dilemma is that a number of people need to be observed in hospital for several days for accurate diagnosis. Several studies have shown that people with GI chest pain who are admitted to hospital and treated as if they were having a heart attack, when in fact they were not, suffer considerable emotional trauma, and some do not recover rapidly.[4]

Costochondritis

This condition is an inflammation or arthritis in the joints between the breast bone (sternum) and the ribs. By passing one's fingers down either side of the breast bone a row of small bumps can be felt. These are the costochondral joints. As with the rib cage, the joints move with every breath. If one of the joints becomes inflamed, the pain often causes spasm in the muscles of the rib cage. The pain may be felt across the front of the chest and may radiate to the sides. Pressing the costochondral joints will make the tender joint obvious and may cause the pain to radiate around the chest. While the pain can seem similar to angina, the tenderness of the joint clearly distinguishes it as costochondritis.

Anxiety

People with anxiety may experience chest pain. The pain is described as sharp, occurring at the sides of the chest and sometimes in the back. It is likely caused by spasm in the muscles in the rib cage. It lasts only seconds or minutes and usually moves from one area to another. There is no local center of pain or tenderness as found in chest wall pain. Its rapidly changing quality usually distinguishes it from other causes.

Pleurisy

Pleurisy, an inflammation of the pleura (the membrane surrounding the lungs), produces a distinctive pain. The sensitive membrane becomes inflamed in association with infection (e.g., pneumonia) in the lung. Every breath causes the inflamed surfaces to rub, which produces pain. Any deep breath, cough, sneeze, or change of position will aggravate this extremely sharp pain. Although the inflammation may occur anywhere on the lung surface, it is most common at the sides of the chest. The pain often radiates widely over the chest.

Trauma

Trauma does not usually present a diagnostic dilemma as the cause is obvious. Broken ribs present a severe pain similar to that of chest wall pain. The pain causes spasm in the muscles of the rib cage causing the pain to radiate. Every breath aggravates pain from broken ribs or bruising of the rib cage muscles.

Myocardial Infarct

Only 3% of all persons experiencing chest pain when they visited their family doctor were actually having a heart attack.[1] These individuals may have had typical angina in the past or silent heart attacks with no pain. The pain caused by myocardial infarct is not relieved by rest, change of position, or use of drugs like nitroglycerine. It lasts longer than 15 to 30 minutes and usually the sufferer looks pale, feels sweaty and unwell, often with nausea and vomiting. Feelings of discomfort, restlessness, shortness of breath, and anxiety are common.

Anyone with these symptoms should be given one adult ASA and be transported to a medical facility immediately. Heart attacks are caused by blood clots which block the coronary arteries that transport blood to the heart muscle. The larger the clot and the longer the heart muscle is deprived of blood and oxygen, the more it will be permanently damaged. Taking an ASA tablet within minutes of the onset of a cardiac chest pain has been shown to benefit heart attack sufferers by reducing the size of the clot.[5] Thrombolytic therapy (injection of drugs to dissolve a clot usually given in the emergency room of a hospital) stops clot formation and may open up blocked blood vessels.[6] The benefits of thrombolytic therapy decline within 3 hours of the onset of chest pain. After 6 hours, no benefit is seen.

Sometimes when a blood clot forms in a coronary artery the change in blood flow affects the "electrical" system in the heart, causing the heart to beat too slowly or too rapidly or even to stop. When this happens the victim suffers sudden collapse, has no pulse, and stops breathing. In some situations the heart is so severely affected that nothing further can be done. However, in many situations, by initiating cardiac resuscitation procedures the patient can survive and, with thrombolytic therapy and rehabilitation, live many more productive years. The possibility of saving lives is a good reason for the general population to learn acute cardiac resuscitation and to maintain their skills. There is evidence that the more people there are with these skills in a community, the more lives saved.

Pulmonary Embolism

A blood clot to the lung is a rare but important cause of chest pain. This pain is of varying quality, can be associated with sweating, pallor, and shortness of breath, and is usually not associated with chest wall tenderness. It should be thought of in anyone with calf tenderness or in women on oral contraceptives, especially smokers and those over 36 years of age.

Other Causes of Chest Pain

There are other rare causes of chest pain that account for 10% of people presenting to their family doctor. Most of the causes, like shingles, have characteristics that distinguish them from cardiac pain.

RECOMMENDATIONS

People should be familiar with the descriptions of the common causes of chest pain. Any person suffering symptoms that suggest a heart attack should immediately be given one adult ASA (325 mg) and transported to a medical facility. Thrombolytic therapy should be given within 3 hours of the onset of chest pain. Everyone should be skilled in acute cardiac resuscitation so that persons suffering a cardiac arrest may be saved.

RECOMMENDATION OF OTHERS

The above recommendations for the management of infarct-like chest pain conform with those of a number of national and international organizations with specific interest in heart problems, such as the Canadian Heart and Stroke Foundation.

REFERENCES

1. A Report from ASPN. An exploratory report of chest pain in primary care. JABFP 1990;3(3): 143–150.

2. Craven MA, Waterfall W. The esophagus as a source of noncardiac chest pain. Can Fam Physician 1988;34:663–668.

3.   Young AJ, McMahon LF, Stross JK. Prediction rules for patients suspected of myocardial infarction. Applying guidelines in community hospitals. Arch Intern Med 1987;147:1219–1222.

4.   Ockene IS, Shay MJ, Alpert JS, et al. Unexplained chest pain in patients with normal coronary arteriograms: a follow up study of functional status. N Engl J Med 1980;303:1249–1252.

5.   Cairns JA, Gent M, Singer J, et al. Aspirin, sulfinpyrazone, or both in unstable angina. N Engl J Med 1985;313:1369–1375.

6.   Basinski A, Naylor CD. Aspirin and fibrinolysis. Lancet 1988;ii:1188–1189.

Physician-Patient Partnership Paper

Patient_____

Chart I.D. _____

Physician _____

The Question: Should I consider a heart problem as the cause of my chest pain?

Information about current health, past health, and family health relevant to the question:

Medical Evidence:

Recommendation: If the pain meets the criteria of a myocardial infarct, take an ASA and seek immediate medical attention. If there is tenderness to touch or increased pain on movement, manage as a musculoskeletal problem. If uncertain, seek medical advice.

Advantages	*Disadvantages*
• decrease anxiety	• create anxiety
• decrease unnecessary investigation	• could lead to delay in treatment
• save lives	

Effect of recommendation on feelings, beliefs, values of self and family:

Physician-patient partnership decision   Date _____

Follow-up plan:

16.5 CHOLESTEROL TESTING

Since heart and vascular conditions are common causes of illness and death in the developed countries, there is great interest in preventing these problems. Elevated cholesterol is one of five risk factors known to predict heart disease.[1] The other four are diabetes, high blood pressure, obesity with a sedentary life style, and smoking, the last being the strongest preventable factor. Although obesity and cholesterol are the weakest of these predictors, cholesterol receives a disproportionate amount of media attention. Public beliefs about cholesterol influence what people eat and what drugs they take, making cholesterol of interest to industries wishing to promote views that favor the use of their products. The result is an ongoing controversy in the media about the importance of cholesterol and confusion among physicians about what steps should be taken to determine who has elevated cholesterol and who would benefit from diet and/or drugs to lower cholesterol.

Evidence of Benefit from Cholesterol Lowering

Few well-designed studies have been carried out to determine if lowering the fat content of a diet reduces the rate of heart disease or death from heart or blood vessel problems. The few large studies, the longest of which ran for 8 years, have failed to show any benefit from lowering the fat content of the diet.[2] Drawing conclusions from these studies might be premature, as it is known that the incidence of heart disease is highest in countries with high dietary fat (usually greater than 40%), such as Scotland, and lower in countries with low-fat diets. Most experts agree that the diet of choice is one with less than 30% of total calories derived from fat.

Drugs studied for cholesterol-lowering effects in large well-designed trials include gemfibrozil,[3] clofibrate,[4] cholestyramine,[5] colestipol,[6] simvastatin,[7] and pravastatin.[8] The trials on the first three drugs demonstrated up to 29% lowering of the number of heart attacks or heart problems. The death rate from heart disease was lower in those given the drugs than in those in the control group. However, when the results were examined for deaths from any cause, those receiving the drugs had the same mortality rates as those not receiving the drugs. For reasons that remain unclear, more people in the treatment groups died from cancer, violent death, and suicide than in the nontreatment groups. These deaths cancelled the benefit of the lower death rates from heart disease, resulting in no overall benefit to taking these drugs.

In 1994, a large Scandinavian trial demonstrated that women and men between the ages of 55 and 75 who had suffered a heart attack or chest pain from heart vessel disease benefited from taking simvastatin if their blood cholesterol was higher than 5.5 mmol/L. This finding was the first to show a benefit in not only reducing the heart attack rate but also the overall death rate in those taking simvastatin compared to those receiving a placebo.[7]

In 1995, a second large study, now known as the West Scotland trial, found that a significant number of men had their rate of heart attacks and deaths reduced by taking pravastatin. All these men had a serum cholesterol level over 7.0 mmol/L at the beginning of the study. All were in good health at the beginning of the study and had no prior heart or blood vessel problems.[7]

RECOMMENDATION

Everyone should lower the fat content of their diet to less than 30% of total calories. At present, there is no evidence that healthy men or women, other than men aged 45 to 65 years, will benefit from cholesterol testing or lowering.

Men between 45 and 65 years, with no symptoms of heart or blood vessel disease should have their cholesterol tested at age 45, and if normal, again in 5 to 10 years. If the result is high (> 6.5 mmol/L), a trial of diet and exercise should be undertaken. If the result remains high, the use of pravastatin to lower the cholesterol to below 5.5 should be considered.

Discussion between physician and patient will be required in those who have other cardiac risk factors. Men and women 55 to 75 who have suffered a heart attack or have developed angina should have cholesterol testing. These individuals should be tested about one month after the development of their symptoms and then treated with simvastatin if their cholesterol is greater than 5.5 mmol/L.

There is at present no evidence to show that the various statin drugs are interchangeable.

RECOMMENDATION OF OTHERS

The Canadian Task Force on the Periodic Health Examination made its recommendations prior to the Scandinavian and West Scotland studies being reported. It recommends that only men 45 to 65 with at least one risk factor should have their cholesterol tested, and gives this recommendation a "C", given the lack of evidence at the time to support more aggressive approaches. It did not recommend any other age or sex group be tested unless other risk factors indicated a need.

The U.S. Preventive Services Task force recommends men aged 35 to 65 undergo periodic cholesterol testing, as a "B" recommendation.

REFERENCES

1.   Neaton JD, Wentworth D. Serum cholesterol, blood pressure, cigarette smoking and death from coronary heart disease. Overall findings and differences by age for 316,099 white men. Multiple risk factor intervention trial group. Arch Int Med 1992;152:56–64.

2.   Frick MH, Elo O, Haapa K, et al. Helsinki Heart Study: primary prevention trial with gemfibrozil in middle-aged men with dyslipidemia. Safety of treatment, changes in risk factors, and incidence of coronary heart disease. N Engl J Med 1987;317:1237–1245.

3.   Report from the Committee of Principle Investigators. A co-operative trial in the primary prevention of ischemic heart disease using clofibrate. Br Heart J 1978;40:1069–1118.

4.   The Lipid Research Clinics Coronary Primary Prevention trial results: 1. Reduction in incidence of coronary heart disease. JAMA 1984;251:351–364.

5.   Dorr AE, Gunderson K, Schneider JC, et al. Colestipol hydrochloride in hypercholesterolemic patients—effect on serum cholesterol and mortality. J Chronic Dis 1978;31:5–14.

6.   Scandinavian Simvastatin Survival Study. Randomized trial of cholesterol lowering in 4444 patients with coronary heart disease. Lancet 1994;344(8934):1383–1389.

7.   Shepherd J, Cobb SM, Ford I, et al. Prevention of coronary heart disease with pravastatin in men with hypercholesterolemia. West of Scotland Coronary Prevention Group. New Engl J Med 1995; 333(20):1301–1307.

Physician-Patient Partnership Paper

Patient _____

Chart I.D. _____

Physician _____

The Question: Should I have a cholesterol test?

Information about current health, past health, and family health relevant to the question:

Medical Evidence:

Recommendation: Healthy men between 45 and 65 should have cholesterol tests every 5 to 10 years depending on the level. If cholesterol is greater than 6.5 mmol/L, treatment should be considered. Men and women 55 to 75, after a cardiac event, should have their cholesterol tested, and if greater than 5.5 mmol/L, should consider therapy.

Advantages
- increased life expectancy for men 45–65 if cholesterol lowered to < 6.5
- men and women aged 55–75 after heart trouble with cholesterol > 5.5 benefit from simvastatin

Disadvantages
- adverse effect from being labeled
- imposes lifestyle change
- some drugs identified as more harmful than beneficial

Effect of recommendation on feelings, beliefs, values of self and family:

Physician-patient partnership decision   Date _____

Follow-up plan:

CHAPTER 17

Physician-Patient Partnership Papers for Cancer Detection

17.1 BREAST CANCER

Breast cancer is the third most common cause of death in women and the most common cause of death from cancer in Canadian women.[1] The risk of breast cancer is increased by a family history of breast cancer and increasing age.[2,3]

The three methods for detection of breast cancer include breast self-examination, manual breast examination by physician or nurse, and mammography (x-ray) of the breast. Early detection is perceived to improve outcome.

Breast Self-Examination

Breast self-examination (BSE) is widely promoted. Many women complain of feeling concerned and anxious for several days prior to doing the examination, are concerned about what they feel, and worry for 2 or 3 days after doing the examination. This negative effect on quality of life can not be justified in the absence of evidence of benefit. A number of trials to determine if early detection of breast cancer by BSE and early treatment prolong life expectancy have conflicting and unclear results.[4-9] Studies may find longer life expectancy because the cancer is detected at an earlier stage in its natural history, and not because life expectancy is actually improved (lead time bias). A recent non-RCT suggests that specific components of BSE done correctly may reduce the risk of death from breast cancer.[10]

Manual Examination of the Breasts by a Physician or Nurse

There have been no studies on the benefits of manual examination of the breasts alone. Every study has looked at mammography and manual examination. Thus, it is impossible to separate the benefits. Given the precision of mammography and the fact that it detects much smaller masses than manual examination, it is likely that most of the benefit of early detection comes from mammography.

Mammography

The original study showing the benefits of mammography was carried out in the 1960s by the Health Insurance Plan (HIP) of New York. It demonstrated that lives were saved in women aged 50 to 60 who underwent a biannual mammogram when compared to women who did not.[11] More recently, a Swedish and a Canadian trial both found that manual breast examination and mammography every 1 or 2 years for women aged 50 to 69 resulted in significantly improved life expectancy.[3,12]

The original HIP study did not demonstrate any benefit from manual examination and mammography for women aged 40 to 50.[12] The Swedish and Canadian trials' results were similar.[13] Breast cancer in premenopausal women behaves differently and responds less well to treatment.

RECOMMENDATION

There is no clear evidence of benefit for early detection by BSE. Some women may find BSE reassuring. The decision of women who wish to discontinue BSE should be supported.

Women aged 50 to 69 should be aware of the benefits of manual examination and mammography. Women under the age of 50 should understand that current evidence does not support mammography.[14] There is no clear evidence that manual examination by physician or nurse alone is a beneficial preventive strategy.

RECOMMENDATION OF OTHERS

The Canadian Task Force on the Periodic Health Examination gives an "A" recommendation to women aged 50 to 69 undergoing annual manual examination and mammographic examination. Although the evidence for benefit of annual over biannual examination is unclear, the Task Force supports annual examination. It gives a "D" recommendation to women under 50 having mammography and gives a "C" recommendation to BSE at any age.

The U.S. Preventive Services Task Force gives an "A" recommendation to women aged 50 to 69 undergoing annual or biannual mammographic screening alone. It states the role of manual examination is unclear and claims insufficient evidence to recommend screening women aged 40 to 49. It does not recommend BSE.

REFERENCES

1.   Statistics Canada. Cancer in Canada. Health Reports 1992;4 (Suppl 8): Catalogue no. 82-0038512, Ottawa.

2.   Hall J, Lee MK, Newman B, et al. Linkage of early onset familial breast cancer to chromosome 17q21. Science 1990;250:1684–1689.

3.   Miller AB, Bains CJ, To T, et al. Canadian National Breast Screening Study: 2. Breast cancer detection and death rates among women aged 50 to 59 years. Can Med Assoc J 1992;147:1477–1488.

4.   Canadian Task Force on the Periodic Health Examination. The periodic health examination: 2. 1985 [update]. Can Med Assoc J 1986;134:724–729.

5.   Greenwald P, Nasca PC, Lawrence CE, et al. Estimated effect of breast self-examination and routine physical examinations on breast cancer mortality. N Engl J Med 1978;299:271–273.

6.   Huguley CM, Brown RL. The value of breast self-examination. Cancer 1981;47:989–995.

7.   Mant D, Vessey MP, Neil A, et al. Breast self-examination and breast cancer stage at diagnosis. Br J Cancer 1987;55:207–211.

8.   Smith EM, Francis AM, Polissar L. The effect of breast self-exam practices and physician examinations on extent of disease at diagnosis. Prev Med 1980;9:409–417.

9.   Philip J, Harris WG, Flaherty C, et al. Breast self-examination: Clinical results from a population based prospective study. Br J Cancer 1984;50:7–12.

10.   Bart JH, Miller AB, et al. Effect of breast self-examination techniques on the risk of death from breast cancer. Can Med Assoc J 1997;157:1205–1212.

11.   Shapiro S, Venet W, Strax P, et al. Selection, follow-up, and analysis of the Health Insurance Plan Study: A randomized trial with breast cancer screening. National Cancer Institute Monograph no. 67,1985, NIH publication No. 85-2713. Department of Health and Human Services.

12. Nystrom L, Rutqvist LE, Wall S, et al. Breast cancer screening with mammography: Overview of Swedish randomized trials. Lancet 1993;341:973–978.

13. Shapiro S, Venet W, Strax P, et al. Ten to fourteen year effect of screening on breast cancer mortality. J Natl Cancer Inst 1982;69:349–355.

14. Miller AB, Bains CJ, To T, et al. Canadian National Breast Screening Study:1. Breast cancer detection and death rates among women aged 40 to 49 years. Can Med Assoc J 1992;147:1459–1476.

Physician-Patient Partnership Paper

Patient_____

Chart I.D. _____

Physician _____

The Question: Should I do breast self-examination each month? Should I have annual mammograms under age 50 or from age 50 to 69?

Information about current health, past health, and family health relevant to the question:

Medical Evidence:

Recommendation: Breast self-examination is not recommended. Screening mammography is recommended for all women aged 50 to 69, but not for women under the age of 50.

Advantages
- mammography reduces mortality rates in women aged 50 to 69
- self-examination and manual examination may reassure some women

Disadvantages
- no clear benefit from BSE
- screening mammography causes anxiety, can be painful, has no benefit for women under 50
- BSE and mammography may result in false positives which require further procedures, or false negatives which incorrectly reassure

Effect of recommendation on feelings, beliefs, values of self and family:

Physician-patient partnership decision   Date _____

Follow-up plan:

17.2   Cervical Cancer

Cervical cancer is rare in the developed countries when compared to lung or breast cancer. In Canada, it is the 11th most common cause of death from cancer in women, with approximately 400 Canadians dying from the disease each year. The natural history of cancer of the cervix is not fully understood. In most cases there is a long interval (between 10 and 25 years) between the first abnormal cells appearing on the cervix to the development of serious disease. Treatment of the disease in its early stages by removal of some or all of the affected cervix is very effective. Women who have never had sexual intercourse are at very low risk for this cancer. If all women who have been sexually active participated in a recommended screening program no women need die of cancer of the cervix.

The Pap Smear

The Papanicolaou smear (Pap smear) is a test where a sample is taken from the cervix using a specially shaped wooden spatula and brush. Because blood and inflammatory effects interfere with the quality of the smear, the test must be done when the woman is not menstruating and is best done in the first one to two weeks after a period and in the absence of a vaginal infection. The material taken from the cervix is preserved and examined under a microscope for cells that show characteristics that could become cancer. False positive results are dealt with by repeating the test, and if abnormal cells continue to be found, the cervix can be examined by colposcopy, a method of examining the cervix under magnification. The Pap test may miss up to 25% of the abnormal cells that are present on the surface of the cervix. False positive and false negative tests are not a major problem because of the long interval between the first appearance of abnormal cells and the development of serious disease.

The risk of missing abnormal cells is dealt with by repeating the test annually for up to three years, reducing the rate of false negative tests from 25% to less than 2%. Only half the women who have abnormal cells on the first test continue to have abnormal cells on subsequent tests.[1-6] Pap smears done as infrequently as once every 5 years are likely to detect up to 90% of cervical cancer at a stage when it can be effectively treated.

Recommendation

All women should have regular Pap smears after becoming sexually active. Current evidence suggests two or three annual Pap smears, followed by a test every 2 or 3 years till age 70. If the woman appears to have above-average risk of cancer e.g., dysplasia on a previous Pap smear, or condylomata (genital warts), then the test may be done more frequently.

Recommendations of Others

The Canadian Task Force on the Periodic Health Examination has modified the recommended frequency for Pap smears three times in the past 15 years. The present recommendation is for all women to undergo two annual Pap smears when they become sexually active, and then every 3 years if these tests are negative, until age 70. In a woman with a history of normal Pap smears, the development of abnormal cells after the age of 70 would be unlikely to reduce life expectancy.

The Canadian Task Force gives the Pap smear a "B" recommendation since there is no randomized controlled trial demonstrating benefit. Such a trial is not likely given the huge numbers required and the need for at least 30 years follow-up.

The U.S. Preventive Services Task Force recommends all sexually active women undergo two annual Pap smears and then be tested once every 1 to 3 years at her and her physician's discretion. Other countries have similar policies with no firm evidence regarding the optimum frequency of screening.

References

1. Boyes DA, Morrison B, Knox EG, et al. A cohort study of cervical screening in British Columbia. Clin Invest Med 1982;5:1–29.

2. Hakama M. Effect of population screening for carcinoma of the uterine cervix in Finland. Maturitas 1985;7:3–10.

3. Lynge E, Poll P. Incidence of cervical cancer following a negative smear. A cohort study from Maribo county, Denmark. Am J Epidemiol 1986;124:345–352.

4. Clark EA, Anderson TW. Does screening by Pap smears help prevent cervical cancer? Lancet 1979; ii(8132):1–4.

5. Stenkvist B, Bergstrom R, Eklund G, et al. Papanicolaou smear screening and cervical cancer. What can you expect? JAMA 1984;252:1423–1426.

6. van der Graaf Y, Zielhuis GA, Peer PGM, et al. The effectiveness of cervical screening: a population based case-control study. J Clin Epidemiol 1988;41:21–26.

Physician-Patient Partnership Paper

Patient _____

Chart I.D. _____

Physician _____

The Question: Should I have a Pap smear to detect cancer of the cervix? How frequently should I have a Pap smear?

Information about current health, past health, and family health relevant to the question:

Medical Evidence:

Recommendation: All women should have two annual Pap smears after becoming sexually active and then every 3 years until age 70.

Advantages	*Disadvantages*
• simple test	• unpleasant procedure
• inexpensive	• only possible when not menstruating
• prevents cancer by detection at precancer or early stage	• has high false negative rate
• if every woman followed the recommendations, the disease would not be lethal	• false positives lead to more tests

Effect of recommendation on feelings, beliefs, values of self and family:

Physician-patient partnership decision   Date _____

Follow-up plan:

17.3 PROSTATE CANCER

There have been suggestions that early detection of prostate cancer in men over 50 could prevent the serious consequences of the disease. Widespread testing for prostate cancer has led to more cases being detected, suggesting an "epidemic," yet there is no evidence of increasing mortality from prostate cancer.[1]

The natural history of prostate cancer is not well understood. At autopsy, 20% of men aged 50, 40% of men aged 80, and up to 90% of men aged 90 have prostate cancer. Most affected men (85%) are unaware that they have the disease. It rarely progresses to cause symptoms or death. Only 7 to 8% of men have an aggressive cancer which spreads extensively and leads to death within 1 to 3 years. The remaining 8% of men develop symptoms and the cancer spreads to bone or other organs, but they appear to respond to hormone and other types of therapy and usually survive for years. There is no effective method at the time of diagnosis to predict which course the disease will take.

Digital Rectal Examination (DRE)

This is the traditional test for early detection of prostate cancer. However, the test is highly inaccurate at an early stage of cancer development. The DRE has no role as a screening test for early detection of prostate cancer.[2]

Transrectal Ultrasound (TRUS)

This test identifies tumors or irregularities in the prostate gland. The procedure is expensive and its interpretation is dependent on the skill of the individual performing the test. There is a high rate of false positives that require biopsy to increase confidence that cancer is not present. The test is not recommended as a screening test in men who have no symptoms.[3]

Prostate Specific Antigen (PSA)

This test also generates a high false positive rate which then necessitates a biopsy.[2,4–9] It does not predict the cancer's speed of development. Some studies have found that most men who have positive PSA tests do not go on to develop any symptoms.[10] Once cancer is detected, usual treatment is removal of the prostate and possibly hormones and radiotherapy.[11,12] Prostatectomy carries a number of serious risks including a 1% mortality rate from the operation, 7% risk of complete incontinence (inability to control the urine), 27% risk of partial incontinence, and a 32% risk of impotence (inability to get an erection). A further 12% go on to develop a narrowing of the urinary passage, and 12% suffer some trauma to their large intestine.[11]

Subjecting the 85% of men with prostate cancer who are unlikely to experience any symptoms to prostatectomy is not justifiable. The PSA test presents medicine with a dilemma. It offers early detection of a potentially serious illness but leads to therapies that are more likely to cause harm than good. It has been suggested by ethicists and the Canadian Task Force on the Periodic Health Examination that any man without prostate symptoms who wishes a PSA test should sign an informed consent form indicating that he understands that this test and its sequelae may cause more harm than benefit.

RECOMMENDATION

Rectal examination and transrectal ultrasound tests do not have enough accuracy to be effective screening tests for prostate cancer in asymptomatic men. The PSA test detects most prostate cancers, but has a high false positive rate. Even when cancer is detected early by PSA there is no way of predicting its natural history. Treatment by removing the prostate gland has serious complications. Since 85% of prostate cancers have a relatively harmless course, early detection and radical treatment cannot be justified. Checking healthy men for cancer of the prostate with a PSA test is likely to cause more harm than benefit and is not recommended.

RECOMMENDATION OF OTHERS

The Canadian Task Force on the Periodic Health Examination does not recommend rectal examination or transrectal ultrasound in persons without symptoms. The Task Force gives PSA testing a "D" recommendation on the evidence that the test does more harm than good in asymptomatic men. The U.S. Preventive Services Task Force states there is insufficient evidence to recommend transrectal ultrasound or PSA tests.

REFERENCES

1.   The Canadian Task Force on the Periodic Health Examination. The Canadian Guide to Clinical Preventive Health Care. Ottawa: Minister of Supply and Services, 1994.812.

2.   Mettlin C, Lee F, Drago J, et al. The American Cancer Society national prostate cancer detection project: Findings of the detection of early prostate cancer in 2425 men. Cancer 1991;67:2949–2958.

3.   Watanabe H, Date S, Ohe H, et al. A survey of three thousand examinations by transrectal ultrasonography. Prostate 1980;158:85–90.

4.   Chadwick DJ, Kemple T, Astly JP, et al. Pilot study of screening for prostate cancer in general practice. Lancet 1991;338:613–616.

5.   Brawer MK, Chetner MP, Beatie J, et al. Screening for prostatic carcinoma with prostatic specific antigen. J Urol 1992;147:841–845.

6.   Gustafsson O, Norming U, Almgard LE, et al. Diagnostic methods in the detection of prostate cancer: A study of a randomly selected population of 2400 men. J Urol 1992;148:1827–1831.

7.   Muschenheim F, Omarbasha B, Kardijan PM, et al. Screening for carcinoma of the prostate with prostate specific antigen. Ann Clin Lab Sci 1991;21(6):371–380.

8.   Labrie F, Dupont A, Suburu R, et al. Serum prostate specific antigen as a prescreening test for prostate cancer. J Urol 1992;147:846–852.

9.   Catalona WJ, Smith DS, Ratliff TL, et al. Detection of organ confined prostate cancer is increased through prostate specific antigen based screening. JAMA 1993;270(8):948–954.

10.   Johansson JE, Adami HO, Andersson SO, et al. High ten-year survival rate in patients with early untreated prostatic cancer. JAMA 1992;267(16):2191–2196.

11.   Wasson JH, Cushman C, Bruskewitz R, et al. A structured literature review of treatment for localized prostate cancer. Arch Fam Med 1993;2:487–493.

12.   Chodak GW, Thisted RA, Gerber GS, et al. Results of conservative management of clinically localized prostate cancer. N Engl J Med 1994;330:242–248.

Physician-Patient Partnership Paper

Patient_____

Chart I.D. _____

Physician _____

The Question: Should I have a rectal examination, transrectal ultrasound, or PSA test to detect cancer of the prostate before it causes symptoms?

Information about current health, past health, and family health relevant to the question:

Medical Evidence:

Recommendation: Rectal examinations, transrectal ultrasound, and PSA tests for early detection of prostate cancer are not recommended in asymptomatic men.

Advantages	*Disadvantages*
DRE	DRE
• inexpensive and simple	• too inaccurate to be of benefit in early detection
TRUS	TRUS
• no clear benefits	• too high a rate of false positive tests
	• high false positive rate
PSA	PSA
• high detection rate of early prostate cancer	• high false positive rate
	• leads to high rate of prostatectomy in men unlikely to suffer adverse effect from cancer
	• prostatectomy carries unacceptable rate of serious complications

Effect of recommendation on feelings, beliefs, values of self and family:

Physician-patient partnership decision   Date _____

Follow-up plan:

17.4   COLON CANCER

In the developed countries, colon cancer is one of the most common forms of cancer in both men and women. A number of factors that increase the risk of colon cancer have been identified. The most important of these is having an immediate family member with this cancer.[1] Other factors that may increase the risk of cancer of the colon include low levels of exercise, high-fat or meat content in the diet, heavy consumption of alcohol, and low intake of vegetables or fiber. The risk is also linked to age. In a 50-year-old, the risk is 18 to 20 times higher than for a 30-year-old, and after age 50 the risk doubles every 7 years. The natural history of the disease is not well understood, but it appears to require several years to progress from polyp to serious disease.

The Digital Rectal Examination (DRE)

The examining finger is very short. The DRE is a poor screening test for colon cancer as it will detect less than 10% of the colorectal cancers in asymptomatic persons.

The Fecal Occult Blood Test (FOBT)

This test involves taking three separate stool samples. The test is very sensitive to the presence of blood or blood-like products, so the patient must avoid consumption of red meat or iron-containing foods for 3 days prior to sampling. Surprisingly large numbers of people will follow these instructions and obtain samples. Ten percent of those taking the test are positive for blood in the stool, when the usual rate of colon cancer is one or two cases in 1000 asymptomatic persons. This high false positive rate means for every one or two people who have cancer, 98 healthy persons must have further testing, usually colonoscopy, which is unpleasant, anxiety provoking, and carries some risk. For those one or two persons who do have colon cancer, there is only a 50% detection rate.[2–6] This poor detection rate is also found in persons at high risk for colon cancer. There is no evidence to support using FOBT.

Sigmoidoscopy

A sigmoidoscope is a metal tube approximately 30 cm (12 inches) long that is inserted into the rectum and can reach 20 to 30 cm into the lower colon. A newer version of the sigmoidoscope is a flexible tube that may reach 10 to 20 cm further. Only the lower 10 to 20% of the colon can be visualized with either instrument. Studies about the accuracy of this test in asymptomatic people have not been done. It is an uncomfortable and unpleasant procedure, which misses a considerable percentage of cancer. It is of little value for screening.[7–10]

Colonoscopy

The colonoscope is an instrument with which the whole colon can be examined. No studies have been done investigating the rate of cancer detection in healthy people undergoing colonoscopy.[11,12] The procedure would not be widely accepted and would likely be impractical as a screening test in people without symptoms.

RECOMMENDATIONS

The poor level of accuracy of the DRE and FOBT suggests that they have no role in early detection of colon cancer. The lack of evaluation of both sigmoidoscopy and colonoscopy in detecting early cancer in asymptomatic people makes it impossible to recommend these tests. It may be that persons at high risk, e.g., persons who have an immediate family member who had colon cancer, should have colonoscopy at some regular interval after the age of 50.

RECOMMENDATIONS OF OTHERS

Different groups disagree on colon cancer screening. Future study results will impact on all groups' conclusions. The Canadian Task Force on the Periodic Health Examination gives FOBT a "D" recommendation meaning that there is some evidence that the procedure does more harm than good. It gives a "C" recommendation to colonoscopy as there is no evidence of harm or benefit from the procedure. It recommends that anyone over the age of 50 with immediate family members who have suffered from colon cancer undergo colonoscopy every 2 years.[12] People at high risk should be aware of the first signs of colon cancer such as blood in their stool or change in their bowel habits and seek the advice of a physician.

The U.S. Preventive Services Task Force has given screening for those over 50, by FOBT or sigmoidoscopy, a "B" recommendation. It is not certain which test should be used, nor the testing interval. It makes a point about the need for informed consent prior to testing. DRE, barium enema (an x-ray of the colon), and colonoscopy are given a "C" recommendation.

REFERENCES

1.   Rozen P, Fireman Z, Figer A, et al. Family history of colorectal cancer as a marker of potential malignancy within a screening program. Cancer 1987;60:248–254.

2.   Mandel JS, Bond JH, Church TR, et al. Reducing mortality from colorectal cancer by screening for fecal occult blood. N Engl J Med 1993;328:1365–1371.

3.   Jensen BM, Kronborg O, Fenger C. Interval cancers in screening with fecal occult blood test for colorectal cancer. Scand J Gastroenterol 1992;27:779–782.

4.   Kewenter J, Bjork S, Haglind E, et al. Screening and rescreening for colorectal cancer. A controlled trial of fecal occult blood testing in 27,700 subjects. Cancer 1988;62:645–651.

5.   Hardcastle JD, Thomas WM, Chamberlain J, et al. Randomized controlled trial of fecal occult blood screening for colorectal cancer. Results of the first 107,349 subjects. Lancet 1989;i:1160–1164.

6.   Winawer SJ, Schottenfeld D, Flehinger BJ. Colorectal cancer screening. J Natl Cancer Inst 1991; 83(4):243–253.

7.   Gilbertson VA, Nelms JM. The prevention of invasive cancer of the rectum. Cancer 1978;41: 1137–1139.

8.   Hertz REL, Deddish MR, Day E. Value of periodic examinations in detecting cancer of the colon and rectum. Postgrad Med 1960;27:290–294.

9.   Selby JV, Friedman GD, Quesenberry CP, et al. A case-control study of screening sigmoidoscopy and mortality from colorectal cancer. N Engl J Med 1992;326:653–657.

10.   Newcomb PA, Norfleet RG, Storer BE, et al. Screening sigmoidoscopy and colorectal cancer mortality. J Natl Cancer Inst 1992;84:1572–1575.

11.   Johnson DA, Gurney MS, Volpe RJ, et al. A prospective study of colonic neoplasms in asymptomatic patients with an age-related risk. Am J Gastroenterol 1990;85:969–974.

12.   Rex DK, Lehman GA, Hawes RH, et al. Screening colonoscopy in asymptomatic average-risk persons with negative fecal occult blood tests. Gastroenterology 1991;100:64–67.

Physician-Patient Partnership Paper

Patient_____

Chart I.D. _____

Physician _____

The Question: Should I have a DRE, FOBT, sigmoidoscopy, or colonoscopy on a regular basis after the age of 50 to detect colon cancer?

Information about current health, past health, and family health relevant to the question:

Medical Evidence:
Recommendation: DRE, FOBT, sigmoidoscopy and colonoscopy are not recommended in healthy people. Persons at high risk, e.g., those with immediate relatives who have suffered cancer of the colon, should have colonoscopy at 2- to 5-year intervals.

Advantages	*Disadvantages*
DRE	
	• low detection rate, unpleasant
FOBT	
• detects 50% of colon cancers	• 10% false positives
• simple and acceptable test	• detects only 50% of cases
• inexpensive	• investigation of false positives required
SIGMOIDOSCOPY	
• better than DRE but still not good screening tool	• unknown benefit in healthy people
	• risk of 1/10,000 bowel perforation
	• visualizes only 20% of colon
	• preparation very unpleasant
COLONOSCOPY	
• best available method for cancer detection	• benefits unknown, not well accepted, with unpleasant preparation
	• risk of bowel perforation, bleeding

Effect of recommendation on feelings, beliefs, values of self and family:

Physician-patient partnership decision   Date _____

Follow-up plan:

CHAPTER 18

Physician-Patient Partnership Papers for Other Common Problems

18.1 SCREENING FOR DIABETES IN ADULTS

A number of symptoms develop with the onset of diabetes (loss of blood sugar control), including excessive thirst, passage of large volumes of urine, weight loss in spite of a good appetite, fatigue, and continuing hunger. If the disease is not treated, symptoms progress to general illness, extreme fatigue, and ultimately loss of consciousness and death. Any person suffering from some of these symptoms needs to have a blood sugar test to rule out the possibility of diabetes. The discussion in this section is confined to performing tests for blood sugar on people who are healthy and have none of the above symptoms. The widely held belief is that early detection of diabetes before any symptoms are present is desirable and beneficial.

There are two types of diabetes mellitus. Type I diabetes almost always occurs in persons under the age of 30 and is most common in young children. Although the cause of Type I diabetes is not fully understood, it seems that these individuals develop an immune reaction to their own pancreatic cells. The pancreas is the organ in the abdomen that, among other things, produces insulin which allows the body to use sugar normally. This immune reaction eventually destroys the insulin-producing pancreatic cells. The individuals become diabetic and must have insulin injections on a regular basis.

Type II diabetics are almost always over the age of 30. Less than 1% of the population under 45 has Type II diabetes, 3.5% between 45 and 64, and 7.55% over 65, making Type II diabetes a common problem in the elderly.[1] Type II diabetics do not produce enough insulin. Their blood sugar can be controlled with diet or with drugs that stimulate insulin production or use. Type II diabetics represent 80 to 90% of all persons who have diabetes. People with parents or siblings who have Type II diabetes have an increased risk of becoming diabetic. Women who have elevated blood sugars during pregnancy have a 30% chance of developing Type II diabetes later in life.

Should Healthy People with No Symptoms of Diabetes Have their Sugar Tested?

It would be desirable to prevent the serious complications of diabetes involving the eyes, vascular system, nervous system, and kidneys through early detection and treatment. Studies carried out over the last 20 years have not demonstrated benefit from early detection, especially in Type II diabetes.[2,3] The best known of these studies demonstrated that careful control of the blood sugars of 1400 Type I diabetics reduced the damage to their eyes over 5 years.[4] There are no studies that show that these results can be applied to Type II diabetics. After 8 years of follow-up of Type II diabetics in a World Health Organization study, no increase in the rate of development of heart or vascular complications was found when the diabetics were compared to nondiabetics of the same age.[5]

RECOMMENDATION

There is no evidence to support blood sugar testing in healthy asymptomatic adults or children.

RECOMMENDATION OF OTHERS

The Canadian Task Force on the Periodic Health Examination gives testing of blood sugars in persons without diabetic symptoms a "D" recommendation on the basis of the inaccuracy of the tests and the lack of evidence of benefit from early detection. The U.S. Preventive Services Task Force recommends that healthy, normal adults with no diabetic symptoms should not undergo blood sugar testing. It does state that discretion should be used in certain high-risk groups.

REFERENCES

1. Young TK, Roos NP, Hammerstrand KM. Estimated burden of diabetes mellitus in Manitoba according to health insurance claims: A pilot study. Can Med Assoc J 1991;144:318–324.

2. Motala AA, Omar MA, Gouws E. High risk of progression to NIDDM in South African Indians with impaired glucose tolerance. Diabetes 1993;42:556–563.

3. Jarret RJ, Keen H, McCartney P. The Whitehall Study: Ten-year follow-up report on men with impaired glucose tolerance with reference to worsening of diabetes and predictors of death. Diabet Med 1984;1:279–283.

4. Welborn TA, Wearne K. Coronary heart disease incidence and cardiovascular mortality in Busselton with reference to glucose and insulin concentrations. Diabetes Care 1979;2:134–160.

5. Bourn D, Mann J. Screening for noninsulin-dependent diabetes mellitus and impaired glucose tolerance in a Dunedin general practice—is it worth it? NZ Med J 1992;105:208–210.

Physician-Patient Partnership Paper

Patient_____

Chart I.D. _____

Physician _____

The Question: Should I have a blood sugar test to detect diabetes before symptoms occur?

Information about current health, past health, and family health relevant to the question:

Medical Evidence:

Recommendation: Blood sugar testing is not recommended in persons who have no symptoms.

Advantages
- early detection of abnormal sugar
- tests are inexpensive and simple

Disadvantages
- tests are not accurate
- early detection provides no benefit
- incorrect labeling is harmful
- testing is anxiety provoking

Effect of recommendation on feelings, beliefs, values of self and family:

Physician-patient partnership decision   Date _____

Follow-up plan:

18.2 LOW BACK PAIN

Low back pain affects about 50% of the population a year and up to 80% of people at some time during their lives.[1–3] Poor physical conditioning, obesity, and heavy lifting all predispose people to low back strain. Studies have not found any specific exercises or preventive steps that reduce the risks of low back strain. There are some indications that being in good physical condition and taking care not to bend or twist while lifting may be helpful.[4]

Is Acute Low Back Pain Serious?

Over 90% of acute low back strains do not require tests or investigations, will improve after 5 days, and completely clear up after 2 or 3 weeks without specific therapy. The most important treatment is to control pain and to continue with daily activities as much as possible. Returning to normal activities even while uncomfortable will shorten the length of the problem by several days and result in a better recovery.[5,6] If the pain radiates from the back down the leg to the ankle or at least below the knee, assessment is advised.

Red flags suggesting that an episode of low back pain requires assessment include a previous history of a cancer, recent unexplained weight loss, back pain that gets worse when resting, and recent trouble with bowel or bladder control. Persons with pain, numbness, or weakness in either leg, and especially in both legs at the same time, should seek medical attention immediately. Persons with AIDS or another disease that could suppress the immune system should be assessed for the possibility of infection in the spine. If there is a chance that infection entered the system from injecting street drugs, assessment is required.[7]

RECOMMENDATION

More than 90% of people with acute low back strain recover within 3 weeks without the need for x-rays or other medical investigation. Recovery is assisted by returning to normal daily activities as quickly as possible, even if some activities are uncomfortable. Although it may be initially uncomfortable, walking can be beneficial. Symptomatic control of pain and reasonable use of heat and cold applied to the back muscles when in spasm may also relieve symptoms.

No specific therapies or exercises during or after the episode of acute low back strain have been demonstrated to be beneficial, and no exercise or educational program has been found which clearly prevents recurrences of acute low back strain.

If after 6 weeks from the onset of the acute low back strain the symptoms have not completely resolved, a further review by a physician is necessary.

OTHER RECOMMENDATIONS

The Agency for Health Care Policy and Research of the National Institute of Health in the United States has developed an excellent set of guidelines for the diagnosis and management of acute low back strain. The above recommendations and discussion are based on those recommendations. The U.S. Preventive Services Task Force gives a "C" recommendation to the use of educational or exercise programs designed to prevent acute low back strain.

REFERENCES

1. Andersson GBJ. The epidemiology of spinal disorders. In: Frymoyer JW, ed. The Adult Spine: Principles and Practice. New York: Raven Press Ltd., 1991;107–146.

2. Cypress BK. Characteristics of physician visits for back symptoms: A national perspective. Am Public Health 1983;73(4):389–395.

3.   Kelsey JL, White AA. Epidemiology and impact of low back pain. Spine 1980;5(2):133–142.

4.   Lahad A, Maiter AD, Berg AO, et al. The effectiveness of four interventions for the prevention of low back pain. JAMA 1994;272:1286–1291.

5.   Nachemeson AL. Newest knowledge of low back pain. A critical look. Clin Orthop 1992;279: 8–20.

6.   Waddell G, Feder G, Lewis M. Systematic reviews of bed rest and advice to stay active for acute low back pain. Br J Gen Prac 1997;47:647–665.

7.   Agency for Health Care Policy and Research, Department of Health and Human Services. Quick reference guide for clinicians. Acute low back problems in adults: Assessment and treatment. Washington D.C. Department of Health and Human Services, 1994. (publication no. 95-0643.)

Physician-Patient Partnership Paper

Patient_____

Chart I.D. _____

Physician _____

The Question: Do I need to see a physician for x-rays or tests for acute low back pain?

Information about current health, past health, and family health relevant to the question:

Medical Evidence:

Recommendation: Simple acute low back pain that does not have any "red flag" characteristics does not require any tests. The most effective treatment is to control pain and resume normal activities as quickly as possible.

Advantages
- rapid return to normal activity speeds recovery
- not having x-rays reduces cost and radiation
- rapid recovery reduces risk of chronic pain

Disadvantages
- rapid mobilization is painful
- lack of medical attention may cause anxiety

Effect of recommendation on feelings, beliefs, values of self and family:

Physician-patient partnership decision   Date _____

Follow-up plan:

18.3   Early Detection of Depression

Depression is one of the most common causes of illness, disability, and death in our society. It is estimated that at least one in five adults will suffer from a serious form of depression during their lifetime.[1] Many people regard depression as a sign of moral weakness, and it has a stigma associated with it which prevents people from easily discussing these problems with a health care provider. Modern understanding of depression relates to brain biochemistry and the altered function of cells in the brain that control affect. During the past 30 years, drugs have become available that alter brain chemistry, allowing those who suffer from depression to lead a normal life. Since treatment can change the natural history of a serious and potentially lethal disease, the same concepts for early detection and intervention which apply to other conditions also apply to depression.

Depression is difficult to identify as there are no blood tests or other physical methods to detect the problem. The diagnosis is a subjective one which utilizes criteria outlined in DSM-IV.[2]

Persons at Risk for Depression

One of the strongest predictors of depression is a previous episode. If a person has had a previous diagnosis of depression they have a 50% chance of a second episode. If they have had two previous episodes they have a 70% chance of recurrence and anyone who has suffered three or more episodes has a 90% chance of recurrence. If there is a family member who has suffered from depression, then the risk is higher. Depression tends to occur more commonly in women and in people under the age of 40. It is common in the postpartum period for women, and tends to occur in people who have serious or debilitating illness. Those who have recently experienced a negative seminal event such as job loss or bereavement are prone to depression. People who are under excessive stress, who are isolated, lack social support, or abuse drugs or alcohol tend to be at higher risk.[1]

Signs of Depression

Depression tends to develop over weeks or months. The early signs of depression may include sleep disturbance, irritability with others, sadness, and loss of interest in such things as friends, family, food, sex, hobbies, reading, or watching television. Many people complain of an inability to concentrate and may begin to make errors in work or at home that would normally never happen. It is often difficult in the early stages to differentiate depression from normal "ups and downs." As the depression becomes more serious, an individual may lose weight, withdraw completely from normal activity, become tearful for no obvious reason, talk of suicide, or state that life is not worth living.

The development of any of these problems in an individual, especially someone with some of the previously mentioned risk factors, should prompt a visit to a physician as soon as possible. The sooner supportive and drug therapy begins, the less time the individual will suffer from depression. Depressed persons are often reluctant to seek help, may resist visiting a physician, and may not want to take prescribed medication. Family and friends can play an important role in the early detection of depression by encouraging the sufferer to seek help and by alerting the physician prior to the visit. Depression comes in many guises and the symptoms can be difficult for the physician to elicit. A number of questionnaires have been developed and tested in physicians' offices to aid detection, but none has been found to be more effective than the physician-patient interview. Work continues in this area.[3–5]

There is a growing tendency to place anyone who has suffered two or more episodes of depression on long-term medication to prevent the high likelihood of recurrence. This is now considered a cost-effective strategy as it can prevent loss of productivity and improve quality of life. Support of friends and family reduces the likelihood of relapse.

RECOMMENDATION

The willingness of the patient's family or friends to report their suspicions of depression to the physician is crucial to its early detection. Their continued support also plays a major role in treatment and the prevention of relapse. Physicians must remain sensitive to the risk factors for depression and maintain an appropriately high index of suspicion. There are no waiting-room questionnaires that have been demonstrated to be practical or effective in early detection of depression.

RECOMMENDATION OF OTHERS

The Canadian Task Force on the Periodic Health Examination does not recommend any questionnaires as none has been demonstrated to be effective in early detection. It does suggest that physician vigilance to symptoms is important. The U.S. Preventive Services Task Force does not recommend that physicians use a questionnaire to detect early depression in their patients. It suggests that clinical sensitivity in looking for depression is very important.

REFERENCES

1.   Shapiro S, German PS, Skinner EA, et al. An experiment to change detection and management of mental morbidity in primary care. Med Care 1987;25:327–339.

2.   Hahn RK, Albers LJ, Reist C. Current Clinical Strategies: Psychiatry. 1997 edition. USA: Current Clinical Strategies Publishing. p.27.

3.   Hoeper EW, Nycz GR, Kessler LG, et al. The usefulness of screening for mental illness. Lancet 1984; i:33–35.

4.   Zung WW, Magill M, Moore JT, et al. Recognition and treatment of depression in a family medicine practice. J Clin Psychiatry 1983;44:3–6.

5.   Magruder-Habib K, Zung WW, Feussner JR. Improving physicians' recognition and treatment of depression in general medical care. Med Care 1990;28(3):239–250.

Physician-Patient Partnership Paper

Patient___ _____

Chart I.D. _____

Physician _____

The Question: What can be done to detect depression early?

Information about current health, past health, and family health relevant to the question:

Medical Evidence:

Recommendation: No tests or questionnaries have been found to be practical in detecting early depression. Family and friends' awareness of the signs and symptoms, seeking medical help, and alerting the physician to their concerns are suggested. Increased awareness of risk factors would help early detection.

Advantages
- early detection reduces risk of serious disability and death
- reduced loss of productivity
- improved quality of life

Disadvantages
- patient often resists assistance
- patient may resist taking medication

Effect of recommendation on feelings, beliefs, values of self and family:

Physician-patient partnership decision   Date _____

Follow-up plan:

18.4   SMOKING CESSATION

Deaths from smoking-related diseases account for 20% of all deaths in Canada each year. These 36,000 preventable deaths account for 271,497 potential life years lost before the age of 75.[1] This makes smoking prevention and smoking cessation a high priority. The ultimate solution to the enormous loss of life and human suffering caused by smoking is to make it socially unacceptable and unattractive, especially to children aged 11 to 13, the average age at which smoking starts.[2]

Benefits of Smoking Cessation

An extensive review conducted by the Surgeon General of the United States in 1990 concluded that there are major benefits to smoking cessation.[3] A smoker's blood contains a high level of carbon monoxide from inhaling smoke saturated with gases, which reduces the blood's capacity to carry oxygen. This reduction in oxygen makes it more likely that in the event of a heart malfunction the heart will beat very irregularly or stop, leading to sudden death. There is an immediate decrease in risk of sudden death from heart attack on the day the smoker stops smoking.

It takes up to 15 years after quitting for a smoker's increased risk of cancer and heart disease to revert to a nonsmoker's risk level. Over 60% of the risk reduction occurs in the first 3 to 5 years after smoking cessation. The health benefits of not smoking should be known and understood by all.

Methods of Smoking Cessation

Tobacco is highly addictive, and most smokers find it difficult to stop smoking.[4] Over 70% of smokers say they would like to stop, and 60% of smokers have attempted to stop at least once. Of those who are successful, 90% quit "cold turkey," often with assistance from family and friends. Twenty percent are successful on their first attempt. Fifty percent of smokers require six attempts to successfully stop.[4] Each unsuccessful attempt to stop smoking brings the smoker closer to success.

Analysis of 39 trials of smoking cessation found that smokers counseled by a physician had a 6% higher success rate than those who did not receive support.[5] Use of nicotine gum or patches with counseling improved results between 4% and 16%.[6] Those who smoked heavily benefited the most from the use of nicotine supplements. Other programs such as smoking cessation groups are of some assistance to those motivated to participate in this type of activity. For those unable to give up their dependence on nicotine, there is a nicotine nasal spray which avoids the harmful effects of tobacco smoke.

RECOMMENDATION

Because of the immediate and long-term health benefits, every smoker should consider stopping. Counseling support from physicians and the use of nicotine gum or patches have been found to significantly improve success rates. A minority of people find that smoking cessation groups are helpful. We would like to make a strong statement about the effects of second-hand smoke, but the evidence is not available.

RECOMMENDATION OF OTHERS

The Canadian Task Force on the Periodic Health Examination and the U.S. Preventive Services Task Force give an "A" recommendation for physicians providing cessation counseling to all smokers and for the use of nicotine gum or patches. The Canadian Task Force gives a

"B" recommendation to individuals' participation in cessation groups and does not find evidence to support counseling individuals about the adverse effects of second-hand smoke.

References

1.   Insight Canada Research. Smoking in Canada: Warnings. Report on the findings of a nationwide survey conducted on behalf of the Canadian Cancer Society, the Heart and Stroke Foundation of Canada and the Canadian Council on Smoking and Health. November 1992:4–21.

2.   Millaa WJ, Hunter L. Household context and youth smoking behavior: prevalence, frequency and tar yield. Can J Public Health 1991;82:83–85.

3.   U.S. Department of Health and Human Services. The health benefits of smoking cessation. Public Health Service, Center for Disease Control, Center for Chronic Disease Prevention and Health Promotion, Office on Smoking and Health, Rockville MD. 1990 DHHS Publication No. (CDC)90–8416.

4.   Kozlowski LT, Wilkinson A, Skinner W, et al. Comparing tobacco cigarette dependence with other drug dependencies. Greater or equal "difficulty quitting" and "urges to use" but less "pleasure" from cigarettes. JAMA 1989;261:898–901.

5.   Kottke TE, Battista RN, DeFriese GH, et al. Attributes of successful smoking cessation interventions in medical practice: A meta-analysis of thirty-nine controlled trials. JAMA 1988;259:2882–2889.

6.   Tang JL, Law M, Wald N. How effective is nicotine replacement therapy in helping people to stop smoking? BMJ 1994;308:21–26.

Physician-Patient Partnership Paper

Patient_____

Chart I.D. _____

Physician _____

The Question: Should I quit smoking? What will help me to stop?

Information about current health, past health, and family health relevant to the question:

Medical Evidence:

Recommendation: There is good evidence of both immediate and long-term benefit from stopping smoking. Aids that assist are repeated attempts, use of nicotine patches or gum, and physician advice and support. Some people benefit from group assistance.

Advantages

- immediate reduction of risk of sudden death
- risk of tobacco-related illness and death returns to average of population after 15 years
- 60% of risk is reduced within the first 3–5 years
- financial savings

Disadvantages

- addiction withdrawal symptoms
- loss of association with break, relaxation, and reward
- associated weight gain of 6–10% in individuals
- psychological struggle

Effect of recommendation on feelings, beliefs, values of self and family:

Physician-patient partnership decision   Date _____

Follow-up plan:

18.5   OSTEOARTHRITIS

Osteoarthritis is a condition best described as wear and tear on the bones and joints of the body. It is among the most common chronic health conditions and is a leading cause of chronic disability.[1] The problem occurs in people in whom there is a strong family history of the condition, or who have sustained trauma to the joints through injury, repetitive occupational or recreational use, or through aging. The cartilage covering the bone surfaces becomes less protective. The bone surface becomes rough and irregular as it deteriorates and when the joint moves, it "grinds" over the surface rather than sliding smoothly.

Initially, osteoarthritis is marked by some stiffness or pain in joints, especially after more-than-usual joint usage (long walks, playing vigorous sports, etc). Joint stiffness is felt after resting and subsides a few minutes after resuming activity. The initial occasional discomfort may slowly develop into a more continuous problem, at times involving swelling and deformity as the joint deteriorates.

Management

Treatment is directed at symptom reduction and improvement in coping, since no treatment has yet been shown to slow the deterioration or alter the long-term course of the problem. Regular aerobic exercise such as walking, cycling, swimming, or water exercise has been shown in many studies to reduce pain and improve physical functioning and mood.[2,3] Leg muscle exercises improve strength and may help to reduce pain.[4,5] Canes and orthotics (customized shoe insoles) may also help to relieve pain.

Nonsteroidal anti-inflammatory drugs (NSAIDs), such as ASA and ibuprofen, and pure pain-relieving drugs such as acetaminophen are widely used. No study has shown that one type of drug is more effective than the other in controlling pain.[6,7] NSAIDs carry the risk of potentially serious complications such as bleeding from the gastrointestinal tract. This is more likely to occur with NSAID use for longer than 1 or 2 weeks, with higher doses, with use in the elderly, and with previous ulcer disease caused by NSAIDs.[8] Since acetaminophen is as effective, much safer, and less expensive than most NSAIDs, it should be tried first, at a maximum dose of 2 extra-strength tablets (500 mg) 4 times daily. If someone at risk for gastrointestinal bleeding must use NSAIDs to control symptoms, then misoprostil can be taken to reduce this risk.[9] Codeine-containing drugs have the disadvantage of causing constipation and mental slowing, and can be habit-forming.

Knee and hip replacement offers relief of pain and restores a good degree of function in most cases. Since these plastic and metal joints last an average of 8 to 10 years with normal use before requiring replacement, the best candidates for this surgery are older persons and those who do not have jobs or leisure activities that put stress on their joints. It is hoped that drugs that prevent or alter the natural history of osteoarthritis will become available in the future.

RECOMMENDATION

The control of osteoarthritic pain is best achieved with 2 extra-strength acetaminophen tablets (500 mg) 4 times daily. Aerobic and strengthening exercises can also be helpful. NSAIDs should be used in low-risk individuals only and always for less than 2 weeks.

REFERENCES

1.   Badely EM, Rasooly I, Webster GK. Relative importance of musculoskeletal disorder as a cause of chronic health problems, disability, and health care utilization: findings from the 1990 Ontario Health Survey. J Rheumatology 1994;21:505–514.

2.   Minor MA, Hewett JE, Webel RR, Anderson SK, Kay DR. Efficacy of physical conditioning exercise in patients with rheumatoid arthritis and osteoarthritis. Arthritis Rheum 1989;32:1396–1405.

3.   Kovar PA, Allengrante JP, MacKenzie R, et al. Supervised fitness walking in patients with osteoarthritis of the knee. A randomized controlled trial. Ann Intern Med 1992;116:529–534.

4.   Chamberlain MA, Care G, Harfield B. Physiotherapy in osteoarthritis of the knees: a controlled trial of hospital vs. home exercises. Int Rehab Med 1982;4:101–106.

5.   Fisher NM, Gresham G, Pendergast DR. Effects of a quantitative progressive rehabilitation program applied unilaterally to the osteoarthritic knee. Arch Phys Med Rehabil 1993;74:1319–1326.

6.   Bradly JD, Brandt KD, Katz BP, et al. Comparison of an anti-inflammatory dose of ibuprofen, an analgesic dose of ibuprofen, and acetaminophen in treatment of patients with osteoarthritis of the knee. N Engl J Med 1991;325:87–91.

7.   Doyle DV, Dieppe PA, Scott J, Huskisson EC. An articular index for the assessment of osteoarthritis. Ann Rheum Dis 1981;40:75–78.

8.   Singh G, Ramey DR, Marfield D, Fries JF. Comparative toxicity of nonsteroidal anti-inflammatory agents. Pharmacol Ther 1994;62:175–191.

9.   Silverstein FE, Graham DY, Senior JR, et al. Misoprostil reduces serious gastrointestinal complications in patients with rheumatoid arthritis receiving nonsteroidal anti-inflammatory drugs: a randomized double blind placebo-controlled trial. Ann Intern Med 1995;123:241–249.

Physician-Patient Partnership Paper

Patient _____

Chart I.D. _____

Physician _____

The Question: Should I take NSAIDs or acetominophen for my osteoarthritis?

Information about current health, past health, and family health relevant to the question:

Medical Evidence:

There is no evidence of any benefit from taking NSAIDs compared to acetaminophen 1000 mg four times daily.

Advantages of NSAIDs	*Disadvantages of NSAIDs*
• relieve acute inflammation	• not very effective for pain
• come in long-acting form	• irritate the stomach
	• can lead to bleeding from gastrointestinal tract
	• have other serious side effects
	• can be expensive

Effect of recommendation on feelings, beliefs, values of self and family:

Physician-patient partnership decision   Date _____

Follow-up plan:

18.6   HEADACHE

Between 70 and 80% of adults report experiencing a headache at some time, but less than half consult a physician about it.[1,2] Headaches are the reason for about 1.5% of visits to family and general practice, and about half of these are new headaches. Most of these people (71%) suffer from tension headaches or mixed tension and vascular headaches.[3]

Tension Headaches

Tension headaches are caused by the very thin layer of muscles beneath the scalp becoming "tight" or going into spasm. These muscles run from the base of the skull at the back of the neck, over the top of the head and attach to the skull above the eyebrows. Contraction of these muscles causes a headache which feels like a "band" around the head, a tightness over the top of the head, or a pain radiating up from the neck. The muscles in the neck and scalp are often tense and are tender to touch. These headaches are often related to stress and fatigue, and usually respond to simple remedies like the application of heat or cold, massage, and acetaminophen.

Mixed Tension and Vascular Headaches

Mixed tension and vascular headaches tend to be more severe than tension headaches, but have similar causes and respond to similar treatment. Once individuals have been reassured that the headaches do not indicate a serious problem in the brain, they may often be able to control the severity of the headaches, so that 50% of sufferers report their headaches as insignificant within 1 year.[3]

Classic Migraine Headaches

Classic migraine headaches occur in 13% of persons presenting to their physician with headache. The classic migraine headache is usually preceded by an aura which may consist of reduced vision in one eye, flashing lights, hearing changes, unusual smells, or a numbness or tingling sensation on the face or upper body. The aura is usually repetitive, recurring in a similar way before each headache, and disappearing with the onset of the headache. The headache usually occurs on one side of the head, is severe and often accompanied by intolerance of bright light, and nausea and vomiting. It usually lasts between 3 and 8 hours. These headaches may be prevented with drugs that dilate the blood vessels when taken at the first sign of the aura. There are new drugs which, when taken regularly, may reduce or prevent the onset of classic migraine headaches.

Sinus Headaches

Sinus headaches are caused by infection in the cavities above and beside the nose. The sinuses drain into the upper nose cavity. If a cold or allergic irritation of the nose causes swelling of the lining of the nasal passages, these openings may become obstructed and the sinus may become infected. The headache is usually constant and may be aggravated by movement of the head. The patient may have a fever and feel unwell. This headache responds dramatically to use of nasal decongestants 3 or 4 times daily for 2 or 3 days. Antibiotics may become necessary if the decongestants are ineffective.

High Blood Pressure

High blood pressure is rarely the cause of a headache, although many people coming to the doctor attribute their headaches to it. The systolic blood pressure would need to be greater than 200 or 220 for some time and would likely have caused symptoms involving visual problems or neurological problems before causing a headache.

Red Flags

Sixty-seven percent of all visits to physicians for headache are really because the patients are worried about having a serious cause for their headache, such as a tumor. Of 1000 people who seek medical advice for headache, 4.1 will have a serious cause.

A headache requires urgent medical attention if it is accompanied by such neurological symptoms as sudden onset of poor or lost vision, usually in one eye, double vision, or visual disturbance such as flashes of light; the onset of weakness, numbness or tingling sensations in arms, legs, or face; a disturbance of speech, thought processes, hearing or other senses; or a headache which is "the worst pain I have ever experienced."

The cause requiring the most urgent attention is meningitis. Meningitis occurs most frequently in children and adolescents. Its incidence has been significantly reduced by the use of *H. influenzae* vaccine. Meningitis usually comes on rapidly with severe headache and discomfort on attempting to move the neck. Progression from being well to seriously ill can take place within hours. The headache is usually accompanied by high fever, generalized illness with nausea and vomiting, and as time goes on, visual and other neurological problems including numbness in limbs, weakness in arms and legs, or even seizures.

Any suspicion of meningitis should prompt immediate medical attention, as time is crucial in beginning intravenous antibiotic therapy to stop the progress of the infection in the brain.

RECOMMENDATION

Most headaches are related to fatigue, stress, or the triggers that cause migraine. They usually respond to application of heat or cold, exercise, or use of common analgesics like acetaminophen, ASA, or ibuprofen. These headaches require medical attention only if they are causing disability because of frequency or severity. Any headache accompanied by generalized illness or the described neurological symptoms requires medical attention and investigations. Any headache that is the most severe pain ever experienced requires medical attention. Any headache of rapid onset accompanied by high fever and neck pain or stiffness that does not respond to adequate dose of acetaminophen in 20 to 30 minutes requires immediate attention to rule out the possibility of meningitis.

REFERENCES

1.   Waters WE. The Pontyprid headache survey. Headache 1974;14:81–90.

2.   Taylor H, Curran N. The Nuprin Pain Report. New York: Louis Harris and Associates, 1985.5.

3.   Becker L, Iverson DC, Reed FM, et al. Patients with new headaches in primary care. J Fam Pract 1988;27:41–47.

Physician-Patient Partnership Paper

Patient _____

Chart I.D. _____

Physician _____

The Question: Is my headache serious, requiring medical attention?

Information about current health, past health, and family health relevant to the question:

Medical Evidence:

Recommendation: Most headaches are related to fatigue, stress, or migraine triggers and respond to application of heat or cold, exercise, or common analgesics. If any of the characteristics that suggest serious headache are present, seek medical attention immediately.

Suggests headache not serious
- comes and goes within minutes
- described as tightness or band around head
- visual or neurological problems precede headache
- usually responds to simple therapy
- often caused by stress or fatigue
- rarely lasts more than 1 day

Suggests serious headache
- steady severe pain
- often with fever and systemic symptoms that do not respond to an adequate dose of acetaminophen
- neurological symptoms accompany headache
- no specific cause identifiable
- persists over days or weeks

Effect of recommendation on feelings, beliefs, values of self and family:

Physician-patient partnership decision   Date _____

Follow-up plan:

18.7   HORMONE REPLACEMENT THERAPY IN WOMEN

Middle-aged women need to consider the benefits and risks of hormone replacement therapy (HRT) or estrogen replacement therapy (ERT). HRT involves taking both estrogen and progesterone; ERT involves taking estrogen only and is suitable for women who have had their uterus removed and no longer need the progesterone to protect them from uterine cancer.

HRT and ERT relieve menopausal symptoms such as hot flashes and vaginal dryness. For the woman with significant symptoms, the promise of relief can be an important factor in her decision. For most women with minor symptoms, the decision is not so simple. The medical benefits and risks must be understood. The information that is continually forthcoming makes advice and counseling of women on this subject increasingly complicated and difficult.[1]

Prevention of Osteoporosis and Prevention of Fractures

Studies have demonstrated that ERT stops the process of bone thinning and, after 2 years of therapy, may strengthen the bones.[2–4] This has been found in women taking hormone pills, using hormone patches, or receiving estrogen injections. One study monitored women for 10 years and found a prevention of bone loss over this time period.[5] There is less clear evidence whether hormone replacement prevents hip fractures, which are a primary cause of loss of life and loss of mobility and independence in older women.[6,7] The studies have found that women benefit most in the first 3 to 5 years of taking hormones. The duration of treatment remains unclear. The effect of the added progesterone remains unclear. It appears that stopping therapy in women who have taken hormone replacement for 10 years results in an accelerated loss of bone in the following years. There is no information about the benefits of starting hormones in women over 70.

Bone density studies could be done for the woman who is ambivalent about HRT. The identification of relatively weak bones might play an important role in her decision making. Smoking cessation, weight-bearing exercise, decreased caffeine consumption, and increased intake of calcium and vitamin D in appropriate quantities can all be initiated with or without bone densitometry. A number of studies have been carried out to demonstrate benefits from bone densitometry screening, but none have been able to demonstrate that early detection prevents the problems of fractures later in life. Newer therapies rapidly arriving on the scene may change this situation.

Reducing the Risk of Heart and Vascular Disease

Studies over the past 10 years have consistently found taking ERT reduces the risk of heart and vascular disease in women over the age of 50 by up to 42%.[8] An analysis combining several studies (a meta-analysis) found the risk of heart attack was reduced by 35% and the risk of death from heart disease was reduced by 33% in women taking ERT compared to women who were not.[9] These studies imply a reduction in overall mortality from the hormone replacement therapy. Note that these studies were carried out on women who did not take any progesterone therapy. Progesterone changes the blood fat content in a way that may increase the risk of heart disease. The benefit of HRT may be similar or somewhat less than ERT but is unknown to date.

Increasing the Risk of Endometrial Cancer

Women who use only estrogen replacement have an increased risk of developing cancer of the endometrium (lining of the uterus). The risk appears to increase with a higher dose and duration of use.[10] The addition of progesterone to the regimen on a regular basis eliminates the risk. In one study, use of progesterone reduced the risk of endometrial cancer to below that of women who took no hormones.[9] All of these studies were on small numbers of women and the methods used are considered weak.

Increasing the Risk of Breast Cancer

The evidence that HRT or ERT increases the risk of breast cancer is conflicting. Meta-analysis of previous studies found a 1.3 times increased risk of breast cancer in women who had used hormone replacement therapy for more than 15 years. Women who had a family history of breast cancer and used hormones had double the risk of breast cancer compared to hormone users with no breast cancer in their family.[9] This single analysis counters three other similar analyses that found no increased risk of breast cancer in women who used hormone replacement therapy.[11–13]

Life Expectancy

The average 50-year-old Caucasian female can expect to live to 82.8 years of age without hormone use, 83.7 years of age if she uses ERT, and 82.9 to 83.8 years of age if she uses HRT. Nothing is known of the quality of this additional time.[9] Women with the greatest risk of coronary heart disease and the lowest risk of breast cancer could have a 41-month gain in life expectancy.[1]

RECOMMENDATION

All middle-aged women should be counseled about the benefits and risks of HRT. Smoking cessation, low-fat and high-fiber nutrition, 1500 mg calcium daily, 400–800 IU vitamin D daily, and moderately strenuous weight-bearing exercise every day are recommended.

RECOMMENDATIONS OF OTHERS

The Canadian Task Force on the Periodic Health Examination gives hormone replacement therapy for prevention of fractures and cardiovascular disease a "B" recommendation, stating that consideration of the risk of breast cancer is necessary. The Task Force gives a "D" recommendation to the use of screening bone densitometry.

The U.S. Task Force on the Use of Preventive Services recommends that all women be counseled about the risks and benefits of HRT. It gives a "C" recommendation for the use of bone densitometry in assessing risk. They advocate that all women should be encouraged to stop smoking, do regular weight-bearing exercises, and consume adequate calcium and vitamin D in their diet.

REFERENCES

1.   Frank J, Evans MF. How does hormone replacement therapy affect the longevity of women with different risk factors? Can Fam Physician 1997;43:1371–1373.

2.   Riis BJ, Thomsen K, Strom V, et al. The effect of percutaneous oestradiol and natural progesterone on postmenopausal bone loss. Am J Obstet Gynecol 1987;156:61–65.

3.   Lindsey R, Hart DM, Clark DM. The minimal effective dose of estrogen for prevention of post menopausal bone loss. Obstet Gynecol 1984;63(6):759–763.

4.   Christianson C, Christensen MS, Transbol I. Bone mass in postmenopausal women after withdrawal of oestrogen/gestagen replacement therapy. Lancet 1981;i(8218):459–461.

5.   Nachtigall LE, Nachtigall RH, Nachtigall RD, et al. Estrogen replacement therapy 1:A ten year prospective study in the relationship to osteoporosis. Obstet Gynecol 1979;53:277–281.

6.   Naessen T, Persson I, Adami HO, et al. Hormone replacement therapy and the risk for the first hip fracture. A prospective population-based cohort study. Ann Intern Med 1990;113:95–103.

7.   Kiel DP, Felson DT, Anderson JJ, et al. Hip fracture and the use of estrogen in postmenopausal women. The Framingham Study. New Engl J Med 1987;317:1169–1174.

8.   Stampfer MJ, Colditz M. Hormone replacement therapy. A quantitative assessment of the epidemiologic evidence. Prev Med 1991;20:47–63.

9.   Grady D, Rubin SM, Pettiti DB, et al. Hormone therapy to prevent disease and prolong life in postmenopausal women. Ann Intern Med 1992;117(12):1016–1037.

10.   Gambrell RD, Massey FM, Castaneda TA, et al. Use of the progestogen challenge test to reduce the risk of endometrial cancer. Obstet Gynecol 1980;55(6):732–738.

11.   Steinburg KK, Thacker SB, Smith SJ, et al. A meta-analysis of the effect of estrogen replacement therapy on the risk of breast cancer. JAMA 1991;265(15):1985–1990.

12.   Armstrong BK. Oestrogen therapy after the menopause—boon or bane? Med J Australia 1988; 148:213–214.

13.   Dupont WD, Page DL. Menopausal estrogen replacement therapy and breast cancer. Arch Intern Med 1991;151:67–72.

Physician-Patient Partnership Paper

Patient_____

Chart I.D. _____

Physician _____

The Question: Should I take hormone replacement therapy?

Information about current health, past health, and family health relevant to the question:

Medical Evidence:

Recommendation: All middle-aged women should consider the benefits and risks of HRT. The authors encourage smoking cessation and excellent nutrition including low fat, high fiber, 1500 mgm calcium daily and 400–800 IU vitamin D. Daily moderately strenuous weight-bearing exercise is recommended.

Advantages
- reduced risk of cardiovascular disease
- reduced osteoporosis (maybe reduced hip fractures)

Disadvantages
- may increase risk of breast cancer
- cost
- side effects of drugs, including vaginal bleeding, and stomach symptoms requiring investigation

Effect of recommendation on feelings, beliefs, values of self and family:

Physician-patient partnership decision   Date _____

Follow-up plan:

Glossary

Analysis of variance (ANOVA). Analysis of variance allows comparisons between the means of two samples of similar populations with a normal distribution. Usually, a dependent variable is identified and the mean measurements of the samples are compared to the mean of the samples of independent variables. The contribution to variance for each variable can be determined, and tested for statistical significance. If five variables contribute to the lowering of blood pressure in a study, ANOVA can indicate how much each of the variables contributes to overall blood pressure lowering.

Bias. Bias is any factor that sways the mind. If, in reading an x-ray, you already know the radiologist has found a hairline fracture, you will search until you see the fracture. Without this information, you would be less likely to find the fracture. If you know a patient in a trial is in the intervention group, and if you believe in the effectiveness of the intervention, you will behave toward the patient and report on the patient's progress differently than if you were not aware the patient was in the intervention group.

Blinding. Blinding is ensuring that all individuals involved in managing a study are unable to identify which patients are in the control or intervention groups. The blinding of the study participants reduces bias in the results of the study.

Case-control study. A case-control study is conducted retrospectively. The charts of a number of patients with the same illness are assembled and the records of people with similar characteristics, but who do not have the illness or have not received the intervention, are compared. Because of the retrospective method of assembling groups, a case-control study is subject to considerable bias.

Cohort study. In a cohort study, individuals assembled at a similar point in their diagnosis are divided into two groups: those receiving and those not receiving an intervention. Efforts are made to match the groups on important characteristics. The cohort study provides a stronger method than does case-control study since it is prospective. The fact that the groups are not assembled by random allocation means there is risk of bias.

Contamination. Contamination in a trial occurs when the intervention and control groups come into contact, resulting in individuals in the control group behaving similarly to those in the intervention group. This contamination artificially dilutes the effect of the intervention and may lead to a Type II error.

Controlled trial. A controlled trial is the comparison between a group receiving medical intervention and a group not receiving the intervention. If individuals have not been randomly allocated to control and intervention groups, then every effort must be made to ensure the intervention and control groups are similar.

Clinical significance. Clinical significance is the benefit to people receiving an intervention, compared to the control group, being great enough to warrant the intervention. If 5000 persons are enrolled in a trial to assess the benefit of a medication for the common cold and 3% of those receiving the drug reduce the duration of their symptoms by 12 hours, the results are statistically significant, but few people will find the results clinically significant.

Cost-analysis. Cost-analysis compares the financial costs of two or more therapeutic interventions, and does not include quality-of-life or other emotional-cost considerations.

Cost-effectiveness. Cost-effectiveness analysis relates all costs to a single outcome for the purpose of making a comparison. An example is the actual cost of an intervention calculated in terms of the dollar cost per life year saved by the intervention.

Cost-minimization. Cost-minimization analysis is the comparison of two or more interventions to determine which has the lowest cost, usually from a single party's perspective.

Cost-utility. Cost-utility analysis goes one step beyond cost-effectiveness and considers measures of quality of life as well as measures of cost. The outcome of a cost-utility analysis is expressed in the number of "quality life years saved."

Descriptive report. A descriptive report describes a single case or a series of cases of individuals suffering from the same illness. There is no effort to select groups or do more than generate a hypothesis from which more organized trials can be mounted. No clinical conclusions should be drawn from a descriptive report.

Discounting. Discounting, in an economic analysis, means a benefit or saving today is greater than the same benefit or saving occurring in the future. Money spent today with immediate benefit is worth more than the same amount spent on an intervention that will save lives in 25 years.

DOE. A DOE is a study in which the outcomes measured are disease oriented. Such outcomes are usually laboratory centered, such as a blood value.

Double blind. In a double-blind trial, neither the staff nor the patient participating in the trial is aware of whether a participant is in the intervention or the control group.

Dose-response gradient. When a low dose reaches a specific level of benefit, an intermediate dose correspondingly provides greater benefit, and so on. Many interventions also have a therapeutic range below which there is minimal or no effect and above which the toxic side effects of the intervention exceed the benefits, making the intervention more harmful than beneficial.

Efficacy. Efficacy is the measure of the consequences of two or more comparable interventions. The measurement includes both costs and all other impacts of the interventions.

Effectiveness. The effectiveness of a therapeutic intervention is measured by how much it improves health status. Effectiveness does not take into account the difference in cost of two or more comparable interventions.

Empirical data. Empirical data is assembled from observations and clinical experience without any attempt to organize or analyze the observation in a scientific way. It is subject to the biases of both the observer and lack of systematic selection of patients. No clinical conclusions should be based on empirical data.

Factor analysis. Factor analysis is a statistical method of measuring the correlation or relationship between several variables in a study. The report of a factor analysis is a series of ratios of the strength of the relationships existing between variables. Factors analysis is used when developing scoring systems in rating scales.

Gold standard. A gold standard test is as close to 100% specificity and sensitivity as possible. When a test is used as "the gold standard," you need to determine if its characteristics justify use of the term.

Meta-analysis. Meta-analysis is the process of combining compatible study results to draw conclusions about the effectiveness of an intervention. This strategy is useful for several studies with smaller numbers of people and inconclusive results, that used the same or very similar methods. By "merging" the data from the small studies, the "power" of a larger study can assist in drawing firmer conclusions.

Negative predictive value. NPV is the proportion of patients receiving a negative test result in whom the test correctly predicted an absence of disease.

Positive predictive value. PPV is the proportion of patients having a positive test result in which the test correctly predicted a positive diagnosis.

Power calculation. Power calculations are used to estimate the number of study participants required to demonstrate a statistically significant difference between groups. In designing a study, preliminary work is done to estimate the difference in outcome likely between the intervention and control groups. If the projection is a 20% benefit for those receiving the treatment, an estimate can be generated of how many people are needed in the trial to demonstrate statistically significant differences, with 95% confidence that the finding of a difference was not determined by chance alone. The estimate of the difference should be determined in as credible a fashion as possible.

Input. Input is the total cost of implementing a therapeutic intervention. Costs must be accounted for in a way that makes two or more different therapeutic interventions comparable. Input costs are classified into three categories in a health economics analysis: (1) organization and operating costs, including health professional time, health care institution or facility operating and capital costs, or overhead costs; (2) patient costs including direct costs to patients and their families for lost work time, patient and family investment in therapy, and emotional cost; and (3) costs borne externally by the economy (indirect costs) including the cost to employers or governments for illness compensation or lost productivity, or the cost to the entire health care system of implementing a procedure.

Output. Output measures include a comprehensive measure of the results of the therapeutic intervention in economic terms. This includes changes in the individual's physical, social or emotional function resulting from the therapy, the impact on use of health care resources, the impact on the patient's family, and on leisure and work. Quality of life is difficult to quantify yet is an essential parameter in a meaningful economic analysis.

Odds ratio. OR is the ratio of the probability of the occurrence of an event to its nonoccurrence. The formula for the odds ratio can be found in Table 5–2. It is used with case-control studies.

POEM. A POEM is a study in which the outcomes measured are patient oriented. Such outcomes often include quality of life measures.

Randomized trial. The process begins with individuals being assembled at a specific point in time and randomly allocated to two or more groups. Usually, one of the groups is a control group which receives no intervention, and the other group(s) receives one or more therapies. Randomization should distribute the patients into two or more groups where any significant differences between the groups would occur only by chance. The purpose of randomized allocation is to reduce the risk of bias causing one group to be significantly different from the other in an important variable, such as age, smoking, socioeconomic status or gender, that could alter the conclusion of a study.

Allocation is usually carried out from a book of random numbers or from a computer program that generates random numbers. The quality of the randomization is checked by measuring certain significant variables between the groups to discover any differences in the characteristic of individuals in each group.

Relative risk. The RR is the ratio of the risk of disease or death among those exposed compared to those unexposed to the danger. Relative risk may also be calculated in groups exposed to different treatments for the same disease. Relative risk should be calculated from information obtained from randomized controlled and cohort studies. The formula for calculation of RR can be found in Table 5–2.

Sensitivity. The ability of a diagnostic test to identify the presence of disease (formula in Table 2–1).

Specificity. Specificity is the ability of a diagnostic test to identify the absence of disease.

Statistical significance. Statistical significance is the likelihood of a difference between two groups being real. Stating statistical significance in another way, it is the possibility that the difference occurred by chance alone. A 0.05 confidence level suggests that 19 times out of 20 the finding of the difference between the two groups is correct and 1 time in 20 the finding is by chance alone.

Temporal relationship. The longer a beneficial medical intervention occurs the greater one assumes the benefit will be. Using an exercise program as an example, following an effective plan for 10 years should have a greater benefit than 5 years or 2 years.

Transparency. Transparency refers to detailed information provided about the methods and process used in a study. Another researcher should be able to replicate the study with the details provided, and arrive at similar conclusions.

Type I error. A Type I error occurs when a study concludes that there is a difference between two groups when there is no difference. The "*P* value" of a test expresses the chance of a Type I error being made in a study. Thus, a *P* value of 0.05 indicates there is a 1 in 20 chance of a Type I error, or a difference being detected between two groups when there is no true difference. Some have called the Type I error a "cloud" error. The analogy is derived from the idea that one can look out a small window and see only clouds, when in reality, the sky is clear with only one cloud in it. Because of chance and a restricted sample, the conclusion is that it is a cloudy day. This conclusion is different from the one arrived at by those outdoors, as they have seen a much larger section of the sky. Your conclusion differs from reality due to chance and a small sample size.

Type II error. A Type II error is concluding that no difference exists between groups when there is a true difference. A *P* value of 0.05 suggests a 1 in 20 chance of no difference between two groups being detected when there is a real difference. Some call this the "Kool-Aid" error. If this fruit drink made from flavor crystals mixed with water is too dilute, it is difficult to tell the difference between Kool-Aid and water. If you blindly sample the two, especially after eating garlic as a "confounding variable," you conclude both drinks are water when, in fact, they are different. This conclusion is a Type II error because of the undetected differences from the small sample size.

U-Curve response. For any intervention, there is a low dose where no benefit occurs, a dose response gradient, and a point where the toxic effects cancel out the benefits and the dose response gradient becomes negative. For any intervention one can plot benefits against toxic effects and generate a U-curve of overall benefit which should help in determining the optimum dose.

Viewpoint. The viewpoint in an economic analysis identifies the individual or group perspective from which costs and benefits will be analyzed. A good analysis includes the viewpoint of all important players involved in a particular intervention: the health care provider, the consumer, and the payer. Often a significant difference exists between these viewpoints. Judgments and "trade offs" to reconcile the differences are required.

Appendix

Examples of the Application for Numbers Needed to Treat Calculation

Problem	Intervention	What is Being Prevented	Duration of Follow-up	NNT to Prevent Additional Events
1. Screening asymptomatic women age 50–69[1]	Mammograph	Death from breast cancer	9 years	1075
2. Diastolic blood pressure[2]	Antihypertensive drugs	Death, stroke, or myocardial infarction	5.5 years	128
3. Elderly living independently[3]	Comprehensive home geriatric assessment	Admission to nursing home	3 years	17
4. Acute myocardial infarction[4]	Streptokinase and ASA	Death within 2 years	2 years	24

REFERENCES

1.   Nustrom L, Rutquist LE, Wall S, et al. Breast cancer screening with mammography: Overview of Swedish randomized trials. Lancet 1993;341(8851):973–978.

2.   MRC trial of treatment of mild hypertension: Principal results. Medical Research Council Working Party. Brit Med J Cl Res 1985;291(6488):97–104.

3.   Stucu AE, Aronow HU, Steiwer A, et al. A trial of annual in-home comprehensive geriatric assessment for elderly people living in community. New Engl J Med 1995;333:1184–1189.

4.   Randomized trial of intravenous Streptokinase, oral aspirin, both or neither among 17,187 cases of suspected acute myocardial infarction. Scandinavian International Study of Infarct Survival Collaborative Group. Lancet 1988;2(8607):349–360.

Index